T0298953

New Genetics, New Identities

New genetic technologies and their applications in biomedicine have important implications for social identities in contemporary societies. In medicine, new genetics is increasingly important for the identification of health and disease, the imputation of personal and familial risk, and the moral status of those identified as having genetic susceptibility for inherited conditions. There are also consequent transformations in national and ethnic collective identity, and the body and its investigation is potentially transformed by the possibilities of genetic investigations and modifications (including the highly controversial terrains of reproductive technologies and the use of human embryos in biomedical research).

The chapters in this volume, drawn from an international array of authors, address these issues from a variety of national, disciplinary and empirical standpoints. An informative read for postgraduates and professionals in the fields of sociology, social anthropology, science and technology studies, and environmental studies, the chapters comprise empirically based and theoretically informed discussions of key sociological, anthropological, political and ethical issues.

Using the resources of a wide range of social science disciplines to provide a comparative approach to complex issues, this superb collection explores the local and global consequences of the new genetics, and analyses the social implications of these advances for identity formation in a period of rapid social change.

Paul Atkinson is Distinguished Research Professor in Sociology at Cardiff University, where he is Associate Director of the ESRC Centre for Economic and Social Aspects of Genomics. He has published extensively on the sociology of medical knowledge and qualitative research methods. He is Co-editor of the journal *Qualitative Research*. He is an Academician of the Academy of the Social Sciences.

Peter Glasner is Professorial Fellow in the Economic and Social Research Council's Centre for Economic and Social Aspects of Genomics at Cardiff University. He is Co-editor of the journals *New Genetics and Society* and *21st Century Society*. He has a longstanding research interest in genetics, innovation and science policy. He is an Academician of the Academy of Learned Societies in the Social Sciences.

Helen Greenslade is Editorial Assistant for CESAGen's Genetics and Society Book Series. She graduated from Cardiff University with a degree in Italian and Spanish, and holds an MA in European–Latin American Relations from the University of Bradford.

Genetics and Society

Series editors:
Paul Atkinson, *Associate Director of CESAGen, Cardiff University*;
Ruth Chadwick, *Director of CESAGen, Cardiff University*;
Peter Glasner, *Professorial Research Fellow for CESAGen, Cardiff University*;
Brian Wynne, *member of the management team at CESAGen, Lancaster University.*

The books in this series, all based on original research, explore the social, economic and ethical consequences of the new genetic sciences. The series is based in the ESRC's Centre for Economic and Social Aspects of Genomics, the largest UK investment in social-science research on the implications of these innovations. With a mix of research monographs, edited collections, textbooks and a major new handbook, the series will be a major contribution to the social analysis of new agricultural and biomedical technologies.

Forthcoming in the series:

Governing the Transatlantic Conflict over Agricultural Biotechnology (2006)
Contending coalitions, trade liberalisation and standard setting
Joseph Murphy and Les Levidow
978–0–415–37328–9

New Genetics, New Social Formations (2007)
Peter Glasner, Paul Atkinson and Helen Greenslade
978–0–415–39323–2

New Genetics, New Identities (2007)
Paul Atkinson, Peter Glasner and Helen Greenslade
978–0–415–39407–9

The GM Debate (2007)
Risk, politics and public engagement
*Tom Horlick-Jones, John Walls, Gene Rowe, Nick Pidgeon,
Wouter Poortinga, Graham Murdock Tim O'Riordan*
978–0–415–39322–5

Local Cells, Global Science (2007)
Embryonic stem cell research in India
Aditya Bharadwaj and Peter Glasner
978–0–415–39609–7

Growth Cultures (2007)
Life sciences and economic development
Philip Cooke
978–0–415–39223–5

New Genetics, New Identities

Edited by Paul Atkinson, Peter Glasner
and Helen Greenslade

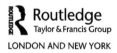
Routledge
Taylor & Francis Group

LONDON AND NEW YORK

First published 2007
by Routledge
2 Park Square, Milton Park, Abingdon, Oxon OX14 4RN

Simultaneously published in the USA and Canada
by Routledge
270 Madison Ave, New York, NY 10016

Routledge is an imprint of the Taylor & Francis Group, an informa business

© 2007 Paul Atkinson and Peter Glasner, editorial content and selection;
individual chapters, their contributors

Typeset in Sabon by
Taylor & Francis Books
Printed and bound in Great Britain by
MPG Books Ltd, Bodmin

British Library Cataloguing in Publication Data
A catalogue record for this book is available from the British Library

Library of Congress Cataloging-in-Publication Data
A catalog record for this book has been requested

ISBN10: 0–415–39407–4   ISBN13: 978–0–415–39407–9 (hbk)
ISBN10: 0–203–96292–3   ISBN13: 978–0–203–96292–3 (ebk)

Contents

List of contributors   vii
Acknowledgements   xi

1   Introduction: new genetic identities?   1
    PAUL ATKINSON AND PETER GLASNER

2   Genetic advocacy groups, science and biovalue: creating
    political economies of hope   11
    CARLOS NOVAS

3   Patients as public in ethics debates: interpreting the role of
    patients' organisations in democracy   28
    ANNEMIEK NELIS, GERARD DE VRIES AND ROB HAGENDIJK

4   From 'scraps and fragments' to 'whole organisms': molecular
    biology, clinical research and post-genomic bodies   44
    SUSAN E. KELLY

5   Fashioning flesh: inclusion, exclusivity and the potential of
    genomics   61
    FIONA K. O'NEILL

6   Mapping origins: race and relatedness in population genetics
    and genetic genealogy   77
    CATHERINE NASH

7   The moral and sentimental work of the clinic: the case of
    genetic syndromes   101
    KATIE FEATHERSTONE, MAGGIE GREGORY AND PAUL ATKINSON

8   Medical classification and the experience of genetic
    haemochromatosis   120
    ADITYA BHARADWAJ, PAUL ATKINSON AND ANGUS CLARKE

9 Towards an anatomy of public engagement with medical
  genetics 139
  ROBERT EVANS, ALEXANDRA PLOWS AND IAN WELSH

10 Genetics, gender and reproductive technologies in Latin
   America 157
   LILIANA ACERO

11 Genomics, social formations and subjectivity 177
   PRIYA VENKATESAN

   Index 191

Contributors

Liliana Acero has been a Research Fellow at the University of Sussex, working on the social and gender impacts of new technologies with a focus on developing countries. She has also been an Associate Visiting Professor at the University of Massachusetts and Brown University. She has taught at various universities and carried out research mainly in Brazil and Chile, and in Argentina, her country of origin.

Aditya Bharadwaj is a lecturer in Medical Sociology at the School of Social and Political Studies, University of Edinburgh. His principal research interest is in the area of new reproductive, genetic and stem cell biotechnologies and their rapid spread in diverse global locales. He was one of the authors of *Risky Relations* (Berg 2006), and is currently completing a monograph, *Conceptions: infertility and technologies of procreation in India*, and co-authoring *Local Cells and Global Science: the proliferation of stem cell technologies in India* (Routledge) with Peter Glasner.

Angus Clarke studied Medical and Natural Sciences at Cambridge and then qualified in Medicine from Oxford University in 1979. As a research registrar in the Department of Medical Genetics in Cardiff, he studied the clinical and molecular genetic aspects of ectodermal dysplasia. Subsequently he worked in clinical genetics and paediatric neurology in Newcastle upon Tyne, developing an interest in Rett syndrome and neuromuscular disorders. He returned to Cardiff in 1989 and is now Professor in Clinical Genetics with particular interests in the social and ethical issues raised by advances in human genetics and in the genetic counselling process. He also teaches and works as a clinician. He represents the Chief Medical Officer for Wales on the Human Genetics Commission. He has co-authored and edited five books, including *Genetics, Society and Clinical Practice* (jointly with Professor Peter Harper). He directs the Cardiff MSc course in Genetic Counselling.

Gerard de Vries is Professor of Philosophy of Science (Chair) at the University of Amsterdam, and Research Fellow at the Scientific Council for

Government Policy in The Hague, the Netherlands. He has published widely on the philosophy of science, science studies, and in particular on the social, cultural and ethical aspects of science and medicine. His books include *Gerede Twijfel: over de rol van de medische ethiek in Nederland* (Amsterdam: Uitgeverij De Balie, 1993), *De Ontwikkeling van Wetenschap: een inleiding in de wetenschapsfilosofie*, third edition (Groningen: Wolters-Noordhoff, 1995), *Zeppelins: over filosofie, technologie, cultuur* (Amsterdam: Van Gennep, 1999), *Wetenschapsfilosofie voor Geesteswetenschappen* (Amsterdam: Amsterdam University Press, 2001, with M. Leezenberg), and *Genetics from Laboratory to Society: the unknown practice of genetic testing* (London: Palgrave/Macmillan, forthcoming, with K. Horstman).

Robert Evans is Lecturer in Sociology at the Cardiff School of Social Sciences and a member of the ESRC Centre for Economic and Social Aspects of Genomics (CESAGen). His first degree in Sociology and Psychology, his MSC in Social Research Methods, and his PhD project that applied the sociology of scientific knowledge to economic modelling and forecasting were all gained at the University of Bath. Robert is the Convenor of Cardiff's MSc in Sociology, Science and Environment, and the Reviews Editor for the journal *Social Studies of Science*.

Katie Featherstone is Senior Lecturer at the School of Nursing and Midwifery, and Research Fellow at CESAGen, both at Cardiff University. A sociologist of medicine, her recent ethnographic work includes an examination of kinship and disclosure in the context of genetic information; the scientific and social construction of a genetic syndrome; and aspects of the randomised controlled trial.

Maggie Gregory is Research Fellow in the Institute of Medical Genetics, School of Medicine at Cardiff University. She is currently working on a project, funded by the Wellcome Trust, on transgenerational family communication about genetic disorders, and is based in CESAGen, Cardiff. Her earlier career background was in social policy development and management in the Civil Service. Her research interests include the social implications of developments in medical genetics and genetic counselling, family narratives, everyday life and the home, the social theory of time and risk, and qualitative research. She is Book Reviews Editor of the journal *Qualitative Research*.

Rob Hagendijk is a sociologist by training and Dean of the International School for Humanities and Social Sciences at the Universiteit van Amsterdam. His research is focused on public controversies about science and technology, public understanding of science, and participation in decision-making. Recent publications include *The Public Understanding* *of Science and Public Participation in Regulated Worlds* (Minerva, 2004) and *Public Deliberation and Governance: engaging with science and technology in contemporary Europe* (2006). With an international team of researchers he completed an EU-funded, eight-country study of public participation in decisions about science and technology.

Susan E. Kelly is Associate Professor in the Department of Sociology, Associate Faculty of the Department of Epidemiology and Clinical Investigation Sciences, and member of the Center for Genetics and Molecular Medicine at the University of Louisville in Louisville, Kentucky. After her doctorate in medical sociology at the University of California, San Francisco, she studied human genetics and history and philosophy of science as a postdoctoral fellow at the Stanford Center for Biomedical Ethics (1995–97). Her research interests include emerging ethics and post-genomic science, sociology of bioethics, and family experiences of childhood genetic conditions.

Catherine Nash is a feminist cultural geographer and Reader in Human Geography in the Department of Geography, Queen Mary, University of London. Her research focuses on geographies of belonging, identity and relatedness. She is currently exploring ideas of ancestry, origins and descent in relation to gender, ethnicity, race and nationhood in popular genealogy and its newly geneticised forms with the support of an ESRC Research Fellowship.

Annemiek Nelis studied Health Science at the University of Maastricht and specialised in Science and Technology Studies. She obtained her PhD from the University of Twente. Her PhD thesis deals with the development of clinical genetics and DNA technology in the Netherlands. She then became a research fellow at the Anglia Polytechnic University in Cambridge. After this, she worked as a lecturer at the Vrije Universiteit and the University of Amsterdam. She is currently deputy director of the Centre for Society and Genomics (CSG) in Nijmegen. CSG is one of the five centres of excellence of the Dutch genomics infrastructure. Her research focuses on the entrenchment of new innovative technologies such as genetics and genomics and on the role of patient organisations in the development of genetic and genomic technologies.

Carlos Novas is a Wellcome Trust Postdoctoral Fellow at the BIOS Centre for the Study of Bioscience, Biomedicine, Biotechnology and Society at the London School of Economics. He is currently working on a project titled 'The political economy of hope: private enterprise, patients' groups and the production of values in the contemporary life sciences'. This project investigates the range of values that are produced in contemporary life science at the intersection between business ethics and bioethics.

Fiona K. O'Neill is completing a PhD based in CESAGen at Lancaster University, on 'Uncanny belongings: ethics and the technologies of fashioning flesh'. Her current work considers human–technology relations with regard to embodiment and the experience of bioethical issues across standard and innovative medicine. She continues to contribute to the ethical debate regarding face transplantation. She has an interest in socio-ethical issues of mental health with particular regard to genetics and neuroscience, especially in the area of autism.

Alexandra Plows is a Research Fellow in the ESRC Centre for Economic and Social Aspects of Genomics (CESAGen) at Cardiff University. She spent several years as an environmental campaigner before taking an MA in social research methods at the University of Wales, Bangor. This was followed by her PhD on UK social movement networks and mobilisations in the 1990s. During her doctoral research she also worked on the ESRC 'Democracy and Participation' programme.

Priya Venkatesan received her PhD in Literature from the University of California, San Diego. Her dissertation dealt with an analysis of scientific texts and communication through literary approaches such as semiotics and narratology. She also holds a MSc in Genetics from the University of California, Davis. She is currently a postdoctoral scholar in the Department of Medicine at Dartmouth Medical School, where she is focusing on molecular biology research into the regulation of beta-globin genes.

Ian Welsh is Senior Lecturer in Sociology at Cardiff University. He has worked theoretically and empirically on scientific and technological change and social movement engagement for more than twenty years. This work includes writings on nuclear power, accidental nuclear war, transport issues and genetically modified crops. He is currently a principal investigator in the ESRC Centre for Economic and Social Aspects of Genomics (CESAGen). His most recent work relates complexity theory to social change and global social movements. His books include *Mobilising Modernity: the nuclear moment* (Routledge, 2000), *Environment and Society in Eastern Europe* (Longman, 1998, ed. with Andrew Tickle) and *Complexity and Social Movements: multitudes on the edge of chaos* (Routledge, 2006, with Graeme Chesters).

Acknowledgements

The support of the Economic and Social Research Council (ESRC) is gratefully acknowledged. The work was part of the programme of the ESRC Research Centre for Economic and Social Aspects of Genomics.

CESAGen

The ESRC Centre for Economic and Social Aspects of Genomics (CESA-Gen) was established in October 2002 as a collaboration between the Universities of Lancaster and Cardiff. CESAGen's main objective is to work with genomic science while investigating the economic and social factors that shape natural knowledge.

The CESAGen Book Series

The General Editors of the series are Paul Atkinson (Cardiff), Ruth Chadwick (Cardiff), Peter Glasner (Cardiff), and Brian Wynne (Lancaster). Between them, the editors enjoy international reputations. Their expertise covers the entire spectrum of relevant research fields – from bioethics and research regulation to environmental politics and risk, to science and technology studies, and to innovative health technologies.

Artist in Residence

Paul Harrison is an artist and researcher with a background and prevailing interest in print, printmaking and publishing. His practice inherently combines the use of traditional print methods and materials with new and developing technologies. The focus of this practice is a developing dialogue and collaboration with laboratory and social scientists as an integral part of a visual investigation into the production of images emerging from new developments in genetics and cell research. He is interested in how this new information is processed and visualised in both a specialist and a public context. He is presently engaged in projects with scientists at the University of Dundee Biocentre, the Human Genetics Unit, MRC,

Edinburgh and Cold Spring Harbor Laboratory (CSHL) New York. He is also artist in residence at the Human Genome Organisation (HUGO) and visiting fellow/artist in residence at the Centre for Economic and Social Aspects of Genomics (CESAGen) at the University of Cardiff. His work can be seen online at http://www.personal.dundee.ac.uk/~plharris (accessed 24 May 2006).

1 Introduction

New genetic identities?

Paul Atkinson and Peter Glasner

Recent innovations in biomedical knowledge – notably in the field of genetics and genomics – have created extraordinarily diverse possibilities in the natural and clinical sciences. At the same time, they have opened up an equally varied range of opportunities and challenges for social and cultural analysts. The translation of social relations and categories into biological terms, and the simultaneous expansion of biomedical engagement with more and more aspects of everyday life, furnish social scientists with a diverse array of topics that demand urgent engagement.

New biomedical technologies repeatedly create the possibility, not merely of new knowledge, but also of new *forms* of knowledge, and new *social formations* too. The latter form the subject-matter of the companion volume to this one (*New Genetics, New Social Formations*, Routledge, 2006). They in turn create the possibility of new bases for *social identity*, individual and collective. The contributions brought together in this volume report empirical research exploring a number of complementary aspects of genetics and the formation of identities.

Identifying the relevance of innovation in biomedical science for self-identity is not in itself a new observation. Recent sociological, anthropological and historical studies of medical or scientific systems, institutions and practices have repeatedly emphasised the intersection of technology, knowledge and identity. The work of Foucault is among the key sources of inspiration here, as is the work of the author who inspired him, Canguilhem. Indeed, Foucault himself mapped out a programme of research on the cultural history of genetic knowledge. In 1969, in his candidacy presentation at the Collège de France (Foucault 1991), he outlined (as he was required to do) a plan for the classes he would deliver. He identified as the central topic 'the knowledge of heredity'. He delineated a programme of work on nineteenth-century thought: '... starting from breeding techniques, on through attempts to improve species, experiments with intensive cultivation, efforts to combat animal and plant epidemics, and culminating in the establishment of a genetics whose birth date can be placed at the beginning of the twentieth century.' While Foucault's own programme remained unrealised in that form, some forty years or so later we find an increasing number of social scientists working on the profound implications of new regimes of genetic knowledge.

The emergence of modern medicine, Foucault had previously argued, was shaped by key changes in technology closely coupled with changes in the institutional context that created a qualitative transformation in medical perception in early nineteenth-century France, a transformation that in turn sets the course for modern biomedical knowledge more generally (Foucault 1972). Canguilhem (1978) also argued that, within the system of knowledge that underpins modern medicine, the 'normal' and the 'pathological' represent two quite distinct frames of reference. One cannot read the pathological off by just extending the range of physiological values beyond the normal limits. Pathology is not merely a quantitative deviation from the norm, but a qualitatively distinct state. David Armstrong, among others, has extended these ideas, suggesting that in the development of twentieth-century medicine we can identify further organising principles that extend the classical, modern notion of 'the clinic' (Armstrong 1983). He identifies, for instance, the mode of knowledge characteristic of 'the dispensary' that takes the medical gaze outwards into the community, that identifies rates and values of normal and unhealthy states. This a medicine, not of individual bodies, but of populations and communities, members of which are susceptible to classification and enumeration. Such a mode of medical understanding puts in question Canguilhem's radical distinction between the normal and the pathological as a universal one, rather than a context-specific characteristic of the classically 'modern' clinic. In more recent years, we have had added to the armamentarium of biomedical knowledge various forms of 'risk' assessment, in which distinctions between the normal and the pathological are transformed once more. The identification of genetic risks or susceptibilities for inherited medical conditions can have far-reaching implications for personal and collective identity.

This intellectual programme has been advanced by a number of authors who discuss the implications of the new medical technologies and their consequences. Rose (2001), for instance, has provided several key discussions of the new politics of 'life itself', developing ideas on 'biovalue' from Waldby (2000), among others. This perspective is also developed in the chapter by Venkatesan in this volume (Chapter 11), in which she reviews contemporary perspectives on biomedical innovation from a Foucauldian perspective.

The scientific and professional identification of risk can create new sources of personal identity and self-perception (cf. Novas and Rose 2000). Risk has the potential to transform the relatively stable categories of normality and pathology. The individual biography and the medical history are given a particular salience, in that *future* physical and mental well-being may be perceived as determined, or at least heavily circumscribed, by genetic fate. We now know a very great deal about the personal and interpersonal implications of major genetic conditions, such as Huntington's

Disease, breast and colorectal cancer, various forms of muscular dystrophy (myotonic, Duchenne, Becker), haemochromatosis and cystic fibrosis. We know that contemporary biomedical research is identifying ever more medical conditions that have at least a genetic component. Physical conditions are now being complemented by psychological conditions in which genetic bases are becoming incriminated: schizophrenia, bipolar disorder, attention deficit disorder and severe depression are all being linked to susceptibility genes. While genetic and environmental interactions are bound to be complex, and further research is certain to result in yet more complexity, the extension of genetic medicine into psychological conditions and behavioural traits will lead to yet further claims for genetic predestination in many domains of everyday life. Genetic susceptibility may not predict actual onset with any certainty, and may not be able to foretell the severity of the condition, but it has the potential to transform our sense of ourselves as embodied social actors, our sense of biographical development, and our sense of personal stability.

There is no doubt that recent developments in genetic science have helped to transform biomedical science and wider medical practice. It would be unwise, however, to attribute all such change exclusively to the scientific revolution occasioned by the human genome project and the exponential growth in post-genomic research. While genomic science has been a significant motor in the development of medical thought, we must not forget that many key idioms of embodiment, health, illness and identity pre-date the genomic revolution itself. Notions of risk clearly pre-date the identification of many illnesses with genetic predispositions – although it is incontrovertible that genetic medicine has given risk a renewed urgency and currency. Likewise, we have not had to wait until the Human Genome Project and its associated activities for the idiom of inheritance to capture inter-generational physical similarities, nor indeed for the observation of familial medical conditions. Genetic medicine sharpens the collective awareness of these phenomena, and has an important impact on medical thought. But it is not a uniquely transformative set of events. It is clear that genetic medicine can contribute to a generic array of risks, susceptibilities and biological bases that impinge on identity, but it is not unique. It is clear that we must avoid genetic exceptionalism.

An increasing emphasis on biological predisposition gives rise to issues of determinism and the *theodicy of suffering*. A genetic basis for ill-health can imply a deterministic or fatalistic attitude towards suffering. Inherited, genetic conditions appear to be a biological form of destiny, an implacably shaping influence on the unfolding of one's life. Inherited predispositions for major conditions such as Huntington's disease can ultimately determine one's personal fate. Likewise, such fate can be transmitted to one's children. Familial conditions and risks can be detected through genetic testing, if suspected. Spontaneous mutations can also give rise to genetic conditions – but are not familial, and are unpredictable. They can, nevertheless, be inexorable in their effects on offspring. The theodicy of genetic illness directs attention towards the search for explanation and meaning. The parents and other family members of affected children can search their own and others' biographies for explanations. Family trees are inspected by family members as much as they are by genetic specialists. Family members engage in mutual surveillance in the attempt to identify the locus of a genetic trait within a kindred, and its mode of transmission (Featherstone *et al.* 2006). There is ample scope for the attribution of blame. Likewise, self-blame and feelings of spoiled identity (stigma) can pervade the everyday world of families with genetic conditions. Family members can therefore seek to interpolate personal and biographical reasons for inherited medical conditions. Genetic risk runs counter to most contemporary discourse concerning personal responsibility and health. We are exhorted to reduce our exposure to health risks, such as poor diet, tobacco or alcohol intake. Environmental factors over which individuals exercise little or no control – such as pollution and industrial hazards – are increasingly brought within a discourse of responsibility and accountability. But genetic risk implies no responsibility. One may act prudently as a consequence: there are decisions to be made concerning reproductive behaviour, and one can elect to have regular check-ups for certain conditions. But there is a sense in which genetic risk – whether inherited or spontaneous – is inexorable. It is in that sense that genetic risk and its surveillance runs orthogonally to the sort of environmental and public surveillance that Armstrong (1983) describes under the auspices of 'the dispensary'. For suffering is again rendered in individualistic terms and in the absence of genetic engineering, the consequences of genetic mutations or deletions are unavoidable. The chapter here by Featherstone *et al.* (Chapter 7) explores some of these issues in the clinical context of dysmorphology – the genetic specialism concerned with abnormal development. Exploring what they call the 'moral and sentimental order' of the genetics clinic, these authors explore how the parents of children with genetically-based problems construct themselves as moral agents, how they construct their own and their children's identities within the realm of normal family life (cf. Voysey Paun 2006). They also explore how the genetics clinic itself functions as a site of moral and identity work, as counsellors and clients co-construct the moral categories of stigma, blame and normality. The clinic provides an arena for the reconstruction of identity for parents and children. In the course of such clinical encounters, the moral and technical work of clinicians themselves is legitimated.

A number of authors have suggested that contemporary genetic technologies necessarily transform the nature of medical knowledge and lead inexorably to a *geneticisation* of medicine and the consequent geneticisation of identity (see, e.g., Hedgecoe 2002). From complementary perspectives, recent accounts of the construction of genetic disease include analyses of the 'expansion' of diagnostic categories and clinical entities. The identification of genetic bases for a widening number of conditions can shift the boundaries of diseases and syndromes previously identified primarily on clinical grounds. The analytic value of the notion of 'geneticisation' in this context has been contested. It is clear that, on the basis of detailed explorations of the practice of contemporary genetic medicine, there is not a simple, reductionist process whereby genetic conditions become 'fixed' as a consequence of diagnostic genetic investigations. It is clear, however, that we must avoid premature closure concerning this point. It is true, as we have already noted, that genetic medicine can give rise to relatively novel phenomena – or can at least give notions like 'risk' renewed and special salience. It is not altogether clear, however, that there is a wholesale process of geneticisation at work that gives rise to exceptional and novel forms of identity. The chapter by Bharadwaj *et al.* (Chapter 8) provides evidence of these processes in the context of genetic haemochromatosis, a potentially serious genetic illness. Bharadwaj and his colleagues show how patients with clinical haemochromatosis seek to develop their own aetiological understandings of the condition, and to extend the clinical definition of their illness to encompass their own lay aetiology. These patients do not, however, present a picture of a 'geneticised' personal identity, in that their symptomatology is what is at stake for them personally, rather than the specifically genetic origin of their condition.

What does lie behind some of these processes of transformation, in so far as they are identifiable, is a renewed form of biological reductionism. To stay with the realm of medicine for a moment, we should note two things. First, genetic medicine is just one of several revolutions in modern medicine that have destabilised previous forms of knowledge, and that have appeared destined to re-draw the biological basis for clinical medicine. We have witnessed such phenomena as the bacteriological, the viral and the immunological revolutions. At just the same time as the genetic revolution, other technologies are giving us profound change in our understanding of neurological function. Stem-cell technologies are often added to the genomic revolution to promise barely conceivable changes in physical treatment, repair and enhancement. We must avoid the kind of technological determinism that implies that each new technology brings in its train wholesale changes in medical knowledge or in the creation of social identities. Older forms of understanding are very durable, and can accommodate novelty, rather than being completely overturned by it.

None the less, forms of biological reductionism, including genetic reductionism, are powerful and productive aspects of contemporary biological, medical and social thought at the beginning of the twenty-first century. The convergences between the biosciences and the social sciences in some quarters – as in behavioural genetics, evolutionary psychology and genetic psychiatry – mean that we face new sources of individual and collective identity, in which biological relatedness and shared biological heritage may play a significant role. As Kelly points out in Chapter 4 of this volume, genetically-based explanations are being extended to an expanded range of behaviours and disorders, while systems biology is simultaneously transforming the nature of those biological explanations.

Post-genomic science and tissue engineering also hold out the possibilities – for good and ill – of human enhancement. Beyond regenerative medicine (such as the replacement of damaged or lost tissues) there is the promise of a 'post-human' condition that projects yet further the enhanced or augmented cyborg. O'Neill's chapter in this volume (Chapter 5) touches on those aspects of genomics. She explores the twin connotations of 'fashioning flesh'. On the one hand, post-genomic science allows us to fashion tissues, in the sense that they can be created and moulded. On the other hand, such crafted tissues can be incorporated within a 'fashion system' whereby the body and its organs are manipulated in accordance with cultural canons of aesthetics and performance.

The biological expression of social identity and difference is not a new phenomenon. The history of biomedical knowledge shows us how the differences of gender have been repeatedly emphasised through the invocation of biomedical categories. At crucial periods of social change, women's social mobility has been challenged by a series of biological and medical counters. The medical opposition to women's academic education, based on various physiological arguments, is but one significant example. The racialised constructions of ethnic difference that have informed eugenic and other interventions have long pre-dated contemporary genetics. While modern geneticists have themselves tended to resist any eugenic interpretations of genetic science, the more general cultural contexts of biomedical understanding have foregrounded the biological basis of social differences. These tendencies are reinforced by aspects of evolutionary psychology and behavioural genetics. The populist versions of these contemporary disciplines, however, clearly reinforce the biological-reductionist view of shared behaviours and individual differences. Taken to its logical extreme, behavioural genetics is likely to attribute an enormous array of ordinary social action to biological substrates, and their persistence to adaptive advantage. The categories of cultural variation are thus in danger of intellectual obliteration in favour of biological reductionism. Now, we are not predicting the demise of the social sciences, nor are we assuming that natural science of the highest quality and integrity will endorse crudely reductionist explanations. We know from the fate of past academic fashions that over-enthusiastic adoption of over-simplified systems of thought are rapidly overturned by the recognition of complexity and variation that escapes simplistic models. Nevertheless, we must be alert to the challenges thrown out by the increasing visibility and currency of reductionist thought.

One need look no further than the success of various forms of popular science that embody genetic ideas about common descent, heritage and ethnicity for evidence of this intellectual trend. To take just one example by way of a starting-point, *The Seven Daughters of Eve* (Sykes 2001) is one popularising work that has taken the available scientific evidence concerning rates of mutation in mitochondrial DNA (as opposed to DNA in the cell nucleus) to construct a conjectural evolutionary path for the descent of large-scale modern populations. Coupled with the 'out-of-Africa' hypothesis of palaeoanthropology, it is plausible to construct lines of descent for contemporary racial populations and trace them back to a very small number of originating ancestors.

A rather different, but comparable, example may be suggested by the popular *Blood of the Vikings* television series and book (Richards 2001). This attempted to marry up our historical knowledge of the patterns of movement of the Viking Norse people round the British Isles with characteristic genetic traits in the modern population. It proves possible to identify 'Viking genes' in those regions that were sites of Viking settlement (such as the Isle of Man), providing evidence of the persistence of distinctive gene pools after many generations. Of course, the identification of 'Vikings' among a British population is hardly controversial, and few, if any, are likely to experience any threat to or transformation in their individual or collective identity. There are, however, other contexts in which the identification of racial origins with a given genetic constitution has some considerable consequence.

This has been amply demonstrated by the work of Parfitt and his collaborators (e.g. Parfitt 2002). He has worked with several groups who self-identify as 'Black Jews'. Their racial identification with Jews is a collective narrative of genetic origins. That narrative has been given added currency, at least in the eyes of the Black Jews themselves, by the identification of genetic markers that they share with Jewish populations elsewhere. For our purposes, it does not matter whether these genetic narratives of shared racial identity are well founded, and whether future investigations will support or modify such claims. What is important is that genetics provides a powerful idiom for the expression of individual and collective identity. The 'facts' of biology furnish a warrant for a particular heritage, and a biologised legitimation for an historical claim. Again, it is important that we do not over-state the unique novelty of the genetic idiom. The rhetoric of biological inheritance and relatedness – couched for instance in the idiom of blood – has long provided a vocabulary of nationality, nobility and purity. The intersection of national and biological identity has been documented in many contexts. The economies of bio-value mean that DNA may be regarded as a national resource, as well as a repository of national characteristics. Whether it be through 'French DNA' (Rabinow 1999) or the molecular patrimony of small nations and indigenous peoples, the genomic revolution has furnished potent resources for the expression of nationhood and shared origins. In the same vein, the idiom of genomics can provide a potent resource for the expression of social differences.

Nash, in this volume, provides us with an important case-study in this area. It is based on a study of the Genographic Project, which is an exercise in mapping human diversity. In Chapter 6 she describes how this programme capitalises on the rise of 'personal interest genomics', which reflects individual social actors' interest in tracing their origins and heritage. This genealogical imagination is also projected onto a collective level. The Genographic Project deploys the rhetoric of understanding the 'human journey', and recapitulates the powerful imagery of 'primitive' origins, a naturalisation of human difference, and a biologised representation of culture. She suggests that racial science still 'haunts' contemporary population genetics. It is clear that the possibility exists, taken in conjunction with other contemporary cultural and political tendencies, for a newly embodied notion of race and nation.

There are, therefore, new genetic narratives that shape the collective identity-work of populations, illness-sufferers and families. They may be variants of existing narratives – of shared heritage, of differentiation and identification, of destiny, of personal blame and stigma. In the foreseeable future such narratives are likely to proliferate, and genetics will continue to be a dominant idiom of expression. The science is likely to be contested, but we shall almost certainly see renewed claims for a biological basis for educational attainment, and for specific abilities. Biological bases for personality, sexual orientation, gender and other sources of personal identity will be claimed with renewed vigour from time to time. Allied to new developments in neuroscience, genomic claims will furnish new sources of social differentiation, esteem and marginalisation. These will be contested issues. Social scientists will undoubtedly resist the biologisation of social categories, while simultaneously studying the claims of its advocates, and charting the ideological uses of biomedical knowledge in ever widening spheres.

New biomedical technologies imply new positioning of various 'publics'. The chapter by Novas in this collection (Chapter 2) discusses how lay, patient advocacy groups operate strategically. Using a case-study of a rare genetic disease, Novas documents how such a group positions itself, how it deploys techniques for becoming knowledgeable, and how its members can become active players in shaping the norms of contemporary science. He shows how the rhetoric of 'hope' is mobilised in the promotion of such groups' interests and aims. Such a case-study amply demonstrates that 'publics' are *made*. They are certainly not homogeneous, and they do not simply exist 'out there'. They are actively produced, and are engaged in producing themselves. This is the theme developed by Nelis *et al.* in Chapter 3, who also discuss 'patients' as 'publics'. They also show that patient organisations do not merely represent patients in scientific and ethical debates, they actively *present* patients. Patienthood is thus a product of the various techniques deployed by the patient groups themselves. Such groups are engaged in the construction of legitimacy for their members and their activities. Novas and Nelis *et al.* thus provide us with complementary views of 'publics' as sources of identity, legitimacy and interest. Evans *et al.* also discuss the construction of 'publics', focusing as they do in Chapter 9 on the proto-politics of oppositional groups. Organised protest movements, such as those opposed to genetically modified crops or stem-cell research, are by no means homogeneous. One cannot attribute to them a generic oppositional stance.

Acero's chapter (Chapter 10) provides an important example of research from Latin America, in which she documents some of the ethical and social issues surrounding the new genetics and reproductive technologies. Hers is a salutary reminder of the fact that analyses of ethics in practice must be sensitive to the local social and economic contexts, and cannot be grounded solely in a 'Western' perspective on science, technology and social transformation. Global science repeatedly confronts more local regimes of ethics, practice and regulation.

It is not only in the sphere of lay populations, patient groups and ethnic communities that new biomedical knowledge engenders new identities. As Evans *et al.* also discuss in their chapter, new scientific paradigms have direct effects on the identities of scientists themselves. There has, for instance, been a general movement within the biomedical sciences away from a reliance on 'wet' (bench) science, to incorporate more and more 'dry' (computational) science. Genomic and post-genomic science, in other words, is increasingly reliant on the new techniques of bioinformatics, as the work of the scientist depends on making sense of vast amounts of sequenced data, statistics and mathematical models. In this process, established ways of working as biologists or clinical scientists must be complemented by new skills and new interdisciplinary teams. Cherished self-identities, say as a 'biochemist' or a 'pharmacologist', are transformed in the process, as new specialisms such as proteomics, pharmacogenomics and nanotechnology emerge. Disciplinary boundaries are shifted, blurred and weakened. Within the intellectual field of biological and medical research we are witnessing major transformations in the division of labour, the moral order of scientific and academic institutions, and the sources of scientific identity.

Kelly's discussion of the material and metaphorical also brings out several of these key developments. She stresses the significance of new cross-disciplinary specialisms, such as the rise of computational methods and systems biology to suggest the emergence of newer forms of biological explanation. The genomic or post-genomic body is thus being transformed, through the metaphors and models used to describe it, and through the material traces used to capture it. The reductionist models of biological explanation are themselves becoming more complex, and in the process encompass more and more strands of paradigm shift in the biological sciences. They repeatedly encroach on the preserve of the social and cultural scientist. In other words, it is not only the boundaries between natural-science disciplines that are shifting or contested. The boundaries between the natural and the cultural are equally subject to challenge. Social scientists are not only forced to examine the consequences of the new science for scientists, clinicians, patients and publics: their own identity may also be at stake.

References

Armstrong, D. (1983) *Political Anatomy of the Body: medical knowledge in Britain in the twentieth century*. Cambridge: Cambridge University Press.

Canguilhem, G. (1978) *On the Normal and the Pathological*. Dordrecht: Reidel.

Featherstone, K., Atkinson, P., Bharadwaj, A. and Clarke, A. (2006) *Risky Relations: family, kinship and the new genetics*. Oxford: Berg.

Foucault, M. (1972) *Birth of the Clinic: an archaeology of the clinical gaze*. London: Tavistock.

—— (1991) 'Politics and the study of discourse', in G. Burchell, C. Gordon and P. Miller (eds), *The Foucault Effect: studies in governmentality*. London: Harvester Wheatsheaf.

Hedgecoe, A. (2002) 'Reinventing diabetes: classification, division, and the geneticization of disease', *New Genetics and Society*, 21 (1): 7–27.

Novas, C. and Rose, N. (2000) 'Genetic risk and the birth of the somatic individual', *Economy and Society*, 29 (4): 485–513.

Parfitt, T. (2002) *The Lost Tribes of Israel: the history of a myth*. London: Weidenfeld and Nicholson.

Rabinow, P. (1999) *French DNA: trouble in purgatory*. Chicago, IL: University of Chicago Press.

Richards, J. (2001) *Blood of the Vikings*. London: Hodder and Stoughton.

Rose, N. (2001) 'The politics of life itself', *Theory, Culture and Society*, 18 (6): 1–30.

Sykes, B. (2001) *The Seven Daughters of Eve*. London: Bantam.

Voysey Paun, M. (2006) *A Constant Burden: the reconstitution of family life*. 2nd edition. Aldershot: Ashgate.

Waldby, C. (2000) *The Visible Human Project*. London: Routledge.

2 Genetic advocacy groups, science and biovalue

Creating political economies of hope[1]

Carlos Novas

The scientific discoveries associated with the new genetics, combined with its anticipatory and promissory discourses of marshalling in a new era of medicine, have fostered the hope that treatments or cures for many human ailments will be found in the near future. While in the past those who were identified as being at risk or diagnosed with a genetic condition may have considered their biological destiny to be an implacable fate, the promissory discourses and rhetoric of the new genetics can serve to foster the hope that their illnesses or those of their loved ones are open to intervention and remediation through the techniques of molecular biology. The publicity encompassing the Human Genome Project, combined with its promotion of the idea that many illnesses have a genetic component, have made it easier for individuals to identify and understand aspects of themselves through the language of genetics and to identify themselves with others who share a genetic condition. Although in the past biologically-based forms of identification have served as a basis for social and political mobilisation, the forms of biosocial collectivism that have emerged in the United States from the 1980s onwards propose that, by becoming involved in biomedical research, patients and their families can work to challenge the conventional authority structures of medicine, science and the state in order to shape the future of their diseases. As a result of these developments, it could be said that, for those affected by a range of genetic conditions, the hope invested in the promises of the new genetics is not only an act of the imagination, but a field of activity that intensifies the hope that the science of the present will bring about treatments or cures in the near future. This movement contributes to a particular form of the capitalisation of life and its investment with significant social meaning. As a way of trying to encapsulate the social, political and economic materiality of the activities of genetic advocacy groups as they try to accelerate the development of treatment or cures, the term *'political economies of hope'* will be developed throughout this chapter.

The principle argument that will be developed in this chapter is that the hopes which genetic advocacy groups invest in science have a materiality that can be considered in political-economic terms. The first part of this argument explores how patients' associations are becoming involved in the governance of disease. Perhaps one of the most significant political dimensions of advocacy groups' involvement in research is that they have become significant authorities alongside physicians and scientists who play a role in the promotion of the health of specific populations. Through becoming knowledgeable about their illnesses, by providing medical information to lay persons and clinicians, through organising and coordinating scientific research efforts, and through their political advocacy efforts, the groups which represent persons affected by genetic conditions exert an influence on how diseases are governed. The second part of my argument makes the claim that, as patients' groups invest in the potential of genomics in order to speed the processes by which cures or therapies are developed, they contribute to a particular form of the capitalisation of life itself by transforming the surfaces and capacities of the body into resources for the production of value. Here I will draw upon the concept of *biovalue* developed by Catherine Waldby (2000). Waldby uses this concept to discuss how biological samples are productive of value in terms of their potential to augment human health and stimulate circuits for the creation of wealth. The third part of my argument makes the claim that, as genetic advocacy groups become involved in the governance of disease and the generation of biovalue, they contribute to the elaboration of novel norms relating to human participation in scientific research and to the distribution of the benefits derived from it. As a way of highlighting some of the features of this political economy, I will develop a case study of a genetic advocacy group known as PXE International.

Hope, genetic advocacy and political economies of hope

How are the activities of patients, their families and the groups which represent them constitutive of political economies that are oriented towards bringing objects of biomedical hope into being? As part of developing an answer to this question, I think it is important to consider first how the experience of illness has become so closely associated with hope in scientific progress. In the context of the contemporary experience of illness, the confidence and hope expressed in scientific progress most prominently exists in situations of desperation or near-hopelessness. In these situations, as Nik Brown (1998) suggests, 'hope serves to designate a vocabulary of survival where survival itself is at stake'. The language of hope draws upon a similar vocabulary to that of scientific discovery: it indicates a willingness to overcome obstacles, transcend limits, and explore new horizons (Brown 1998; Franklin 1997). To have or 'live' in hope means to take an active stance towards the future so that the possibilities inherent in the present may be rendered achievable. Hope can thus structure the lives of individuals or families affected by illness, and since it often exists in relation to despair, is a profoundly emotional domain of experience that is embodied in various ways (Brown 1998; Franklin 1997; Good *et al.* 1990).[2] One form through which hope can be embodied is through the donation of blood or tissue so that science can transform them into techniques or knowledge that can be used to treat or cure.

In the highly contingent and uncertain illness experience of rare diseases where science may represent the only modality for understanding a particular condition (Rabeharisoa 2003), the ability of hope to be constantly renewed, refreshed and adapted, despite setbacks, perhaps goes some way towards explaining its salience. As we learn from the women in Sarah Franklin's ethnographic account of IVF, they constantly have to renew and 'manage their hopes' in response to the failure of this technology if they are to sustain their determination to continue with the arduous treatment cycles. The hopes *embodied* in biomedical science and technology are thoroughly capitalised, as Franklin (1997) draws out. The ingenuity and knowledge that make it possible to lend a 'helping hand' to nature come at a price, in terms of the private costs of IVF treatment and the personal sense of loss that often accompanies its failure. Despite the dual costs which IVF imposes on many women, their investment in the hope offered by this technology, in most instances, transcends the self and is projected on to those who may subsequently benefit from the march of scientific progress. Hope, it could thus be said, is both individual and collective: it ties together personal biographies, collective hopes for a better future, and broader social, economic and political processes.

It is the relational qualities of hope that make it possible to consider studying it in a political economy context. As hope involves an interplay between the present and the future, and requires individual and collective activity to enable its realisation, it is congruent with the formulation of strategies. To enable hope requires the coordination and management of the conduct of individuals and multiples so that a particular future may come into being. The range of processes through which specific futures are envisaged and acted upon in the present to the exclusion of others can be studied sociologically. Within what can be termed the 'sociology of expectations' (Hedgecoe and Martin 2003) the future is considered to be a contested object of social and material action. To shape or secure the future requires the mobilisation of a range of rhetorical, organisational and material resources to create direction and convince others of what the future may bring (Brown *et al.* 2000). As science constitutes one horizon along which potential futures are constructed, genetic advocacy groups, by engaging with scientists and advocating for particular forms of research, treatment modalities and forms of regulation, are actively involved in shaping particular futures to the exclusion of others (Shostak 2004).

One of the ways in which patients' organisations are involved in capitalising their hopes and shaping the future is through the range of their political advocacy efforts. The growth and rising prominence of patients' groups has been documented in recent sociological studies which investigate the dynamics of social movements in the field of health (see Brown and Zavestoski 2004 and Hess 2004 for two recent journal issues dedicated to this topic). These studies highlight how patients' associations help individuals to transform personal experiences of illness into a social problem and a political issue. They further provide instruction on how to mobilise effectively within these domains (Allsop *et al.* 2004; Brown *et al.* 2004; Rose and Novas 2004). Here the successful experiences of particular groups or coalitions can 'spill over' (see Allsop *et al.* 2004; Brown *et al.* 2004; Zavestoski *et al.* 2004), to use a term borrowed from the study of social movements, creating novel templates for subsequent social and political action. The mediation of illness experiences, the creation of collective identities and their political mobilisation can be thought of as one of the distinctive political roles of genetic advocacy groups.

Another sense in which patients' associations are involved in the capitalisation of their hopes is through facilitating the production of scientific knowledge. While patients' organisations have long played an 'auxiliary role' to the medical profession by providing support to those affected by a particular illness (Rabeharisoa 2003; Rapp *et al.* 2002), increasingly they are becoming directly involved in the mobilisation of scientific research communities. Perhaps the template for this new form of disease advocacy 'spilled over' from AIDS activists. As Steven Epstein (1996) documents, AIDS activists were successfully able to form themselves into experts and thus have an impact on the production of knowledge about this illness, influence the design of clinical trials, and shape policies relating to drug regulation. Patients, families and carers, it could be said, have started to play a direct role in governing risks to their health. One of the ways they do this is by forming themselves into experts through reading the relevant medical literature and scientific journals, and accessing the wealth of health-related information on the internet. This type of activity can extend to the mobilisation and coordination of networks of scientists. As the work of Vololona Rabeharisoa and Michel Callon (2004) on the Association Français contre les Myopathies (AFM) indicates, patients' groups can play a key role in directing scientific research through coordinating and funding it in directions that it considers to be strategically important (see also Rabinow 1999). Through directly engaging in the production and funding of scientific knowledge, patients' groups shape the ways in which the new technologies for visualising and knowing vital life processes are assembled and organised to suit particular social and political objectives.

As a way of trying to encapsulate how the political activism of patients' groups contributes to the way in which life itself is increasingly locked into an economy for the generation of health and vitality, the production of wealth and the creation of social norms and values, I will develop a case study of PXE International, a genetic advocacy group which has made a significant impact upon the condition pseudoxanthoma elasticum. This case study draws upon material published by PXE International in its newsletters and website, the articles and speeches written by its founders, and press reports that have appeared about PXE International in the media. While the experience of PXE International is in some ways unique, it bears some resemblance to accounts produced about patients' associations in the United States, France and the United Kingdom (Allsop *et al.* 2004; Gibbon 2005; Rabeharisoa and Callon 2004; Rabinow 1999; Rapp 2003; Rapp *et al.* 2002). The selection of this case study is by no means meant to be representative of the scope and range of activities (or lack thereof) undertaken by genetic advocacy groups in the United States. This case study should be taken as emblematic of how some patients' groups are creating novel templates for social and political advocacy and are engaged in reframing the conventional ways in which scientific research is conducted.

Hope, identity and the governance of genetic diseases

The diagnosis of an illness can often propel individuals and families to identify with others who share a biological condition and to perhaps join or form a genetic advocacy group. In the case of PXE International, the initiation of its founders Patrick and Sharon Terry into the world of genetic advocacy began in 1994 following the diagnosis of their two children, Elizabeth and Ian, with a rare genetic skin disorder known as pseudoxanthoma elasticum (PXE). This disease affects anywhere between one in twenty-five thousand and one in fifty thousand people. It can cause the calcification of the tissues of skin, eyes and arteries, resulting in hardening and loss of elasticity. PXE can lead to sagging skin, central vision loss, and premature death due to the hardening of arteries or gastro-intestinal bleeding.

Following the diagnosis of their children, the Terrys spent considerable time visiting medical libraries, photocopying relevant articles and reading the medical and scientific literature. By engaging in this programme of research, it could be said that the Terrys began to understand their children's condition in the language of bioscience. Drawing upon the work of Paul Rabinow (1996), these forms of biological identification can lead to the formation of ties with other individuals and families who share a genetic condition. As Nikolas Rose and I (Novas and Rose 2000; Rose and Novas 2004) have suggested, these forms of biological identification and affiliation can lead citizens to make demands upon the state and the scientific community. In the case of the Terrys, they decided to become proactive in the governance of their children's illness by founding PXE International in 1995. Based on the range of skills they possessed through having worked in a number of non-profit organisations, they decided to help build up a community that provides support to persons affected by PXE, and that initiates and funds research (Terry 1996; Terry and Terry 2001). They build up this community through using the medium of the internet and by enrolling dermatologists, ophthalmologists and dentists in putting patients into contact with PXE International. In a very short period of time this organisation has been able to build up a network of 59 offices in thirteen countries. This network not only provides support to those affected by PXE and distributes information to clinicians, it also helps to raise considerable funds to support scientific research efforts that are considered to make a difference to the future governance of PXE.

As individuals affected by genetic conditions become knowledgeable about their illnesses, and as identity begins to take on biological colourations, hope can become bound up with the production of scientific truth. In the case of Patrick and Sharon Terry, as they read more about the disease which threatens the health of their children, they started to realise that the available literature did not paint a clear picture of the disease. In the words of the Terrys: 'We desperately hoped that research was underway that would solve this problem quickly ... we clung to the life raft of the promises and possibilities of research. After an extensive survey of the literature, we felt frustrated and disillusioned. To our profound disappointment, we quickly learned that research on PXE was not cohesive enough to constitute a life raft' (Terry and Terry 2001). The Terrys realised not only that there was a scarcity of knowledge about this disease, but that the little research that was being done was not coordinated in any way. At this moment, Sharon Terry recollects, 'We began to scheme about what we would do if managing research on this disease. PXE did not have a central repository for blood or tissue and also needed a large cohort to understand the condition's progression and manifestation' (Terry 2003c). Based on Patrick Terry's experience as a project manager for a construction firm, where he managed the simultaneous installation of the plumbing and electricity, they wondered if the research that needed to be done on the various aspects of PXE could be accelerated by placing it on parallel tracks (Terry 2003c). Towards this end, the Terrys began to contact and meet with scientists who had written on PXE in the peer-reviewed literature. Many of these scientists eventually became part of PXE International's Scientific Advisory Board and helped to develop a strategic plan to fast-track research (see Terry *et al.* 1999). Through engaging in the coordination of scientific research efforts, organisations such as PXE International are becoming involved in the governance of disease.

Before moving on to discuss some of the ways in which PXE International has participated in the governance of PXE, I want draw out some elements of Patrick and Sharon Terry's narrative, since it has a bearing on the qualities of hope and patient-group involvement in research. Hope can involve a critique of existing circumstances and the promotion of visions of what the future can or should be. The enablement of these hopes or visions requires action in the present in order to bring about a desired state of affairs. What often fuels the involvement of genetic advocacy groups in research is a critique of the conventional structure of science. The limits to the pace of scientific progress which Patrick and Sharon Terry identify consist of: the unwillingness of scientists to share samples with one another, resulting in small and redundant collections; limited pools of participants willing to take part in research; competition amongst laboratories; the lack of funding for rare disease research; the career and tenure concerns of scientists; the nature of the scientific publication process; and the lack of proper informed consent procedures. Perhaps the greatest problem which they identify is the lack of coordination and consensus within the research community and the absence of any mechanisms to ensure such coordination and consensus (see Stockdale and Terry 2002). It is within this problem space that the involvement of genetic advocacy groups in research can help to accelerate the pace of scientific progress by creating pools of resources such as biobanks or disease registries that can be distributed simultaneously to laboratories, developing strategic plans to coordinate different elements of research, and by facilitating collaboration amongst laboratories (Stockdale and Terry 2002; Terry 2003b; Terry 2003c; Terry and Boyd 2001; Terry and Terry 2001). It is important to point out that this concern with the rationalisation and acceleration of science is profoundly embodied – it is driven by the hope that science will develop therapies or cures expeditiously, since time is running out for those who are affected by genetic conditions.

PXE International has already made a significant impact upon the acceleration of research efforts and the governance of PXE, by funding and coordinating a number of projects. These projects act upon the future of this disease by contributing to understanding its natural history, pathology and genetic basis. Central to PXE International's ability to coordinate research are a registry of affected persons throughout the world and a blood and tissue bank – of which more later. PXE International has contributed to studies which have made an impact upon the lives of persons affected by PXE. One such study found that women affected by PXE are not at greater risk of having adverse pregnancy outcomes and should therefore not be discouraged from reproduction (Bercovitch *et al.* 2004). PXE International is further involved in contributing to the generation of knowledge about this disease through helping to design, and recruit over 600 individuals to participate in, the largest epidemiological study to date on this illness concerned with characterising its symptoms, their progression, and the effects of lifestyle in influencing its course (PXE International 1998). PXE International has also contributed to attempts to understand the genetic basis of the disease by funding a study which sought to discover a natural mouse model of the disease (PXE International 1996b). It also works closely with and coordinates the research efforts of a number of laboratories in the United States, The Netherlands, South Africa, Belgium, Italy and Hungary to identify the mutations associated with PXE, understand the function of the gene, and examine the cellular biology of PXE. Through initiating, funding and coordinating scientific research, PXE International not only makes an impact upon the future governance of this disease, but also fabricates the social identities of those affected by genetic conditions as active and critical participants in the production of scientific knowledge.

A final way in which PXE International is involved in the governance of disease is through its political advocacy efforts. This organisation shapes the political mobilisation of PXE sufferers by providing information on pending legislation, encouraging individuals to write or speak to their political representatives, and by providing instruction on how best to advocate for persons affected by skin disorders. Many of PXE International's advocacy efforts are directed towards increasing the funding allocated to the National Institutes of Health (NIH). Early on in the development of the organisation, through a congressional letter-writing campaign and the lobbying efforts of Patrick and Sharon Terry in Washington, DC, it was able to influence a borderline NIH grant decision (which did not consider PXE a relevant disease) to fund the work of Dr Charles Boyd to study elastin gene defects in PXE (PXE International 1996c). It is important to point out the organisation does not solely advocate on behalf of PXE, but more broadly for skin diseases in general. It does so by participating and taking active leadership roles in the Coalition of Patient Advocates for Skin Disease Research and the Coalition of Heritable Disorders of Connective Tissue. Its involvement in advocating on behalf of those affected by genetic disease extends to Sharon Terry's election as President and Chief Executive Officer of the Genetic Alliance, a coalition which represents over 600 genetic advocacy groups in the United States. Patrick Terry serves as President of the International Genetic Alliance, which brings together representatives from coalitions of patients' organisations across the world. By taking leadership roles and working within a number of coalitions, Patrick and Sharon Terry are able to influence the ways in which the hopes and promises associated with the new genetics are realised to benefit persons affected by genetic conditions.

Economies of life: generating health, wealth and biovalue

Genetic support groups have long played a role in the governance of disease by providing assistance to those faced with a debilitating condition, by campaigning for their rights in political or social terms, and by seeking to reduce the stigma associated with a genetic condition. While many of those who worked in these organisations no doubt hoped for a day when a cure or therapy would become available, a key difference that can be noted today in organisations such as PXE International is the sheer scale at which they are involved in capitalising these hopes by investing in the potential of the new genetics to understand the molecular basis of disease and to develop treatments or cures. What is significant about these developments is how genetic advocacy groups contribute to furthering the transformation of life into a resource for the generation of value. Of course, advances in the life sciences over the past thirty years have done much to transform the ways in which vital life processes can be manipulated and become generative of what can be termed *biovalue*. This term was introduced by Catherine Waldby (2000) in her study of the Visible Human Project. For Waldby, biovalue refers to the ways in which bodies and tissues derived from the dead are generative of value through enhancing the health and vitality of the living. Using the example of PXE International, I propose to analyse how this organisation contributes to the generation of biovalue along three dimensions: first, in terms of enhancements to human health; second, the potential to generate economic value; and third, the creation of ethical values relating to the production of health and wealth.

PXE International generates biovalue through its attempts to produce health from the biological samples donated by individuals and families affected by PXE. The PXE International Blood and Tissue Bank, established shortly after the formation of this organisation, constitutes just such a resource. This 'biobank' was established so that those affected by PXE would only have to donate their blood or tissue once, rather than donating multiple times to different research projects (PXE International 1996a). The 'biobank' was also established to overcome a problem that often hinders research on rare diseases: the lack of an adequate sample size to conduct statistically informative genetic studies. Since its inception, this biobank has been able to gather 1500 DNA samples, 100 tissues samples, 1000 pedigrees, and epidemiological data on over 600 individuals (Stockdale and Terry 2002). By facilitating the centralised collection and storage of these samples and enabling their simultaneous distribution to researchers whose projects are approved by the PXE International Scientific Advisory Board, the biobank fits into this organisation's objective to accelerate research in an ethically informed manner (Terry and Terry 2001).

The PXE International Blood and Tissue Bank has proved to be a repository of biovalue. In terms of generating potential enhancements to the health of those affected by PXE, the gene was localised on chromosome 16 in 1997 (van Soest *et al.* 1997) and identified in 1999 as the ABCC6/MRP6 gene (Bergen *et al.* 2000; Le Saux *et al.* 2000). Already this discovery has led to significant advances in developing a genetic test for PXE through collaboration with the biotechnology firm Transgenomic (PXE International 2005; Transgenomic 2002). In conjunction with the epidemiological study conducted by PXE International, the discovery of the gene makes it possible to analyse genotype/phenotype relationships. The identification of the gene has made it possible to develop a mouse model that will assist in understanding the molecular pathways of PXE and serve as an experimental site to trial potential therapies (PXE International 2005). However, the discovery of the genetic basis of PXE may not only generate health for those affected by this particular illness, but potentially for those suffering from apparently unrelated disorders. PXE is part of the ABC (ATP-binding cassette) family of genes. This family of genes is responsible for transporting molecules in and out of cells. Understanding the molecular biological pathways related to PXE may shed light on illnesses such as Stargardt disease, cystic fibrosis, Tangier disease and retinitis pigmentosa. More broadly, the molecular pathways of PXE could contribute to understanding age-related macular degeneration and cardiovascular disease – illnesses which affect the health of millions. At the PXE Research Meeting held in 2004, scientists working on diseases which share similar molecular pathways as PXE were invited in order to facilitate the cross-fertilisation of research endeavours (PXE International 2005). The identification of the ABCC6/MRP6 gene is representative of one dimension of biovalue whereby the manipulation of blood and tissue generates knowledge that can ultimately be used to promote human health.

Within contemporary genomics, the very same techniques that are used to generate health can also lead to the creation of wealth. It could be said that the new genetics, by rendering the depths of the body amenable to visualisation, intervention, inscription and calculation, makes it congruent with the production of economic value. What is being accomplished through the contemporary life sciences is a kind of 'flattening' of the vital processes of the body. This not only enables these 'flattened surfaces' to become equivalent with one another at the most basic biological level, but also allows them to be enfolded within processes of capital or social accumulation. In the life sciences, one of the key routes for the enfolding of life itself within networks of economic exchange is through patents. In the case of PXE, a patent has already been granted in relation to methods for diagnosing and treating this condition (Boyd *et al.* 2004; Marshall 2004). As a result of Sharon Terry's scientific contributions in helping to discover the ABCC6/MRP6 gene, she was named as a co-inventor on the patent alongside researchers at the University of Hawaii. As a co-inventor and through negotiations with the University of Hawaii, the rights to the patent were assigned to PXE International (see Fleischer 2001 for details of these negotiations; Terry 2003b) Already, PXE International has a range of non-exclusive licences, exclusive licences, co-exclusive licences, restricted use licences, and various types of benefit-sharing arrangements with a total of nineteen laboratories and eight companies (Terry 2003b). However, the logic that drives this patent licensing strategy is not driven by the imperatives of capital accumulation, but by those of social distribution. The licensing arrangements are seen as a means of helping to promote access to the gene, ensuring that any diagnostic tests developed are affordable, and facilitating the development of treatments. PXE International intends to use some of the revenues generated by the licensing of the gene to subsidise the costs of genetic testing for PXE once it becomes available (Terry 2003b). PXE International is not only engaged in the transformation of vital life processes into resources for the generation of biovalue, but also in the creation of ethical values relating to the production of health and wealth.

Markets, morals and values: reshaping participation in research

As vital life processes are increasingly being penetrated by market relations in order to generate health and wealth, the values, social norms and ethical practices through which treatments or cures are developed is undergoing change. For groups such as PXE International who are interested in accelerating the pace of scientific research, the economic and legal mechanisms associated with the creation of genetic products and services are not considered to be antithetical to their aims, but rather as resources that need to be harnessed in order to benefit individuals affected by genetic conditions. In writing about the discovery of the gene associated with PXE, Patrick Terry notes that in all likelihood it would have been patented by a bio-technology firm or research institute (Terry 2003a). Rather than simply voicing opposition to patenting, Terry suggests that the assignment or acquisition of patent rights by genetic advocacy groups represents a solution to corporate control of genetic material. It can act as a powerful vector for the advancement of 'patient-centric opportunities' through the licensing of patents in such a way that promotes access to it by a large number of researchers and ensuring that any diagnostic tests or treatments developed are accessible and affordable to affected individuals (Stockdale and Terry 2002; Terry 2003a). In an economy where life is being capitalised, genetic advocacy groups have to work to promote a different range of values through which the market can benefit persons affected by genetic conditions.

As lay persons become increasingly involved in the governance of disease, the coordination of scientific research efforts and the establishment of biobanks, it could be argued that they are starting to become significant authorities who shape the discourses, practices and moral economies through which humans participate in research and its benefits are socially distributed. By acting as an obligatory point of passage between donors of biological samples and the scientific research community, genetic advocacy groups such as PXE International occupy a unique terrain on which to shape the ethics of biomedical research. This can take the form of emphasising that human participation in research should be truly informed. In writing about informed consent, the Terrys suggest that scientists often do not have the time, skills or resources to ensure that participants in research are truly informed about its nature and outcomes in a culturally sensitive matter (Terry and Terry 2001). It is claimed that genetic advocacy groups can play a key role here in educating their membership about the nature of the scientific research process. Furthermore, through maintaining disease registries or biobanks, patients' groups can play an important role in helping to protect the anonymity and confidentiality of their membership by acting as a 'firewall' between them and the scientific research community, holding the keys or codes to unlock personally identifiable information. Lay persons can further be involved in reframing ethical discourses and vocabularies. The Terrys argue that humans who become involved in research should not be considered as *research subjects*, but as *participants* in the research process who have a stake in its direction and outcomes (Terry and Terry 2001) Consistent with this approach, the Terrys are interested in a range of mechanisms that would ensure that any benefits derived from scientific research flow in some way back to those who participated in it. Their ethical concerns here are consumer-oriented. As potential consumers of the results of scientific research, genetic advocacy groups such as PXE International are interested in ensuring that genomic technologies and services are affordable and accessible to those who need them most.

Conclusion

Hope, as manifested in contemporary disease advocacy organisations such as PXE International, relates to a field of strategic action in the present to help realise and bring to fruition the multiple potentialities embodied in contemporary science. A key concern of many participants in this political economy is to accelerate the processes by which science is able to develop genetic tests, diagnostic techniques and therapeutic interventions. The hopes expressed by participants in genetic advocacy groups and the varied actions they collectively take to realise their aspirations constitute one of the many horizons where the future is being mapped on to the present. No doubt, as previous investigators have found, many of those who articulate and act upon their hopes in contemporary science tend to be white, middle-class, educated and highly capable of mobilising social networks both in person and through the medium of the internet (Epstein 1996; Rapp 1999; Stockdale and Terry 2002). Through their ability to successfully organise themselves into groups, to mobilise persons, scientific researchers and politicians, and to raise substantial financial resources, these individuals and collectives have shaped a considerable political economy organised around the hope and potential for science to generate treatments or cures. What is significant about these political economies of hope is how patients, their carers, and advocacy groups are starting to play a central role in the governance of disease, are contributing to the transformation of life itself as a resource for the production of health and wealth, and are beginning to introduce new norms into the scientific research enterprise.

By acting upon the world of science in order to shape the future of their diseases, the varied activities of patients' groups has a distinctly political dimension in that that they are starting to play a role in the governance of disease. Considered along one plane, this can encompass a whole range of self-help techniques for becoming knowledgeable about a particular illness – such as reading the relevant medical literature. A second avenue along which patients' associations are starting to play a noteworthy role in the governance of disease is through forming partnerships with scientific researchers in order to facilitate, coordinate and hopefully accelerate research on a specific illness. As can be seen in the case of PXE International, this organisation plays a key role in the governance of pseudoxanthoma elasticum. This has taken form through the provision of information on the disease to both lay persons and clinicians, the establishment of a blood and tissue bank, the collection of epidemiological data, and by facilitating collaboration amongst a consortium of nineteen laboratories. A third dimension along which patients' groups are starting to play a role in the governance of disease is through their political advocacy and campaigning efforts to increase the portions of national budgets allocated to scientific research and to develop legislation which has a positive impact upon the lives of those affected by genetic conditions. In acting upon the science of the present to accomplish their hopes and aspirations, patients and the organisations which represent them now play a vital role in the governance of disease by becoming educated about their illness, by coordinating and managing scientific research efforts, and by advocating politically on behalf of their disease.

The hopes invested by genetic advocacy groups in the potential of contemporary science to understand the underlying molecular basis of disease, to develop genetic tests, and to create novel therapeutic interventions has a substantial economic component. Especially in the case of rare diseases, the funding provided by disease advocacy organisations often supersedes or matches that provided by national governments or the pharmaceutical industry. Of course, it needs to be pointed out that investments in the science of the present to hopefully develop a range of health services in the future can sometimes take place at the expense of meeting the current economic, social or educational needs of those affected by illness (Stockdale 1999; Stockdale and Terry 2002). Considered along another dimension, through investing in the potential of the new genetics, patients' groups are contributing to the transformation of the potentialities inherent in life itself into a resource for the production of health, wealth and a range of ethical values – or, as this chapter has considered it, biovalue. As such, genetic advocacy groups help to support a shift in the legitimating values of science from being predominantly concerned with the production of truth to that of being oriented around the production of health (Rabinow 1996). However, as most students of contemporary genetics are well aware, the production of health is nowadays intimately bound up with the generation of wealth. As the case of PXE demonstrates, the discovery of the genetic basis of this disease holds the potential for augmenting the health of those affected by this genetic disorder – and potentially for all of us – in addition to retaining the capacity to produce wealth through the licensing of the technology which led to the discovery of the gene. PXE International is representative of the complex intersection between health and wealth in specific political economies of hope. What is perhaps of greatest interest for the future is the norms that are being articulated by advocacy groups in relation to the ethical values embedded in the production of science, health and wealth.

As the hopes of patients and their carers are giving rise to a substantial political economy, it is useful to begin to think about what impact they are having on the norms of contemporary science. The commercialisation of science within the university has been well studied in the social science literature (Andrews and Nelkin 2001; Gold 1996; Kenney 1986; Kloppenburg 1988; Krimsky 1991; Shiva 1997; Yoxen 1983). As Paul Rabinow (1996) has pointed out, so far the transformation of the organisational structure of biotechnology firms to mirror that of academia has not been a topic of considerable concern within the social sciences. With the growing social, political and economic significance of genetic advocacy groups, perhaps it is appropriate to begin thinking about their potential for introducing new norms into both of these sectors. As patients' associations start to play a role in organising and managing collaborations between laboratories, they attempt to eliminate competition between them, organise the timely sharing of information amongst them, and place emphasis on making this research public. As participants or 'partners' in the scientific research enterprise who increasingly control access to valuable 'banks' of human blood and tissue, patients' groups are capable of reframing conventional bioethical approaches to the donation and gifting of human body parts. This conventional approach enables human tissue to be gifted or donated for the 'benefit of humanity', whilst simultaneously retaining its value for potential commercial exploitation (Sunder Rajan 2003). Already we are beginning to witness how groups such as PXE International subvert this subtle logic of bioethical appropriation through exercising claims that participants in research should receive some of the benefits derived from the results of scientific research, and that genetic technologies should be made accessible and affordable to those who need them most.

Notes

1 This chapter has benefited from the very generous comments of Nikolas Rose, Cathy Waldby, Ilpo Helen, Sahra Gibbon, Oonagh Corrigan, Elena Novas and Patricia Peña. This research was made possible through postdoctoral fellowships from the ESRC and the Wellcome Trust.
2 Mary-Jo Delvecchio Good and colleagues (Good *et al.* 1990) use the term 'political economy of hope' to link together cancer research and treatment institutions, the patterns of availability and promotion of particular anti-cancer therapies, the search for cures by patients and their families, as well as the norms of disclosure associated with cancer treatment. While their work uses this term, they do not develop it in their paper. They focus predominantly on norms of disclosure of cancer diagnoses and the importance clinicians attach to instilling hope within cancer patients.

References

Allsop, J., Jones, K. and Baggott, R. (2004) 'Health consumer groups in the UK: a new social movement?', *Sociology of Health & Illness*, 26 (6): 737–56.

Andrews, L. and Nelkin, D. (2001) *Body Bazaar: the market for human tissue in the biotechnology age.* New York: Crown Publishers.

Bercovitch, L., Le Roux, T., Terry, S. and Weinstock, M. A. (2004) 'Pregnancy and obstetrical outcomes in pseudoxanthoma elasticum', *British Journal of Dermatology*, 151: 1011–18.

Bergen, A. A. B., Plomp, A. S., Schuurman, E. J., Terry, S., Breuning, M., Dauwerse, H. *et al.* (2000) 'Mutations in ABCC6 cause pseudoxanthoma elasticum', *Nature Genetics*, 25 (2): 228–31.

Boyd, C. D., Csiszar, K., LeSaux, O., Urban, Z. and Terry, S. (2004) 'Methods for diagnosing pseudoxanthoma elasticum', United States Patent No. 6,780,587: Assigned to PXE International and University of Hawaii.

Brown, N. (1998) 'Ordering hope: representations of xenotransplantation: an actor-network account'. Unpublished PhD Dissertation, Lancaster: University of Lancaster.

Brown, N., Rappert, B. and Webster, A. (2000) 'Introducing contested futures: from *looking into* the future to *looking at* the future', in A. Webster, N. Brown and B. Rappert (eds), *Contested Futures: a sociology of prospective techno-science.* Aldershot: Ashgate.

Brown, P. and Zavestoski, S. (2004) 'Social movements in health: an introduction', *Sociology of Health & Illness*, 26 (6): 679–94.

Brown, P., Zavestoski, S., McCormick, S., Mayer, B., Morello-Frosch, R. and Gasior Altman, R. (2004) 'Embodied health movements: new approaches to social movements in health', *Sociology of Health & Illness*, 26 (1): 50–80.

Epstein, S. (1996) *Impure Science: AIDS, activism, and the politics of knowledge.* Berkeley, CA: University of California Press.

Fleischer, M. (2001) 'Patent thyself', *The American Lawyer*, 21 June.

Franklin, S. (1997) *Embodied Progress: a cultural account of assisted conception.* London: Routledge.

Gibbon, S. (2005) 'Community, the commons and commerce; the ownership of BRCA genes and genetic testing', in N. Redclift (ed.), *Contesting Moralities: science, identity and conflict.* London: UCL Press.

Gold, E. R. (1996) *Body Parts: property rights and the ownership of human biological materials.* Washington, DC: Georgetown University Press.

Good, M.-J. D., Good, B., Schaefer, C. and Lind, S. E. (1990) 'American oncology and the discourse on hope', *Culture, Medicine and Psychiatry*, 14 (1): 59–79.

Hedgecoe, A. and Martin, P. (2003) 'The drugs don't work: expectations and the shaping of pharmacogenetics', *Social Studies of Science*, 33 (3): 327–64.

Hess, D. J. (2004) 'Health, the environment and social movements', *Science as Culture*, 13 (4): 421–27.

Kenney, M. (1986) *Biotechnology: the university-industrial complex.* New Haven, CT: Yale University Press.

Kloppenburg, J. R. J. (1988) *First the Seed: the political economy of plant biotechnology, 1492–2000.* Cambridge: Cambridge University Press.

Krimsky, S. (1991) *Biotechnics and Society: the rise of industrial genetics.* New York: Praeger.

Le Saux, O., Urban, Z., Tschuch, C., Csiszar, K., Bacchelli, B., Quaglino, D., Pasquali-Ronchetti, I. M. P. F., Richards, A., Terry, S., Bercovitch, L., de Paepe, A. and Boyd, C. D. (2000) 'Mutations in a gene encoding an ABC transporter cause pseudoxanthoma elasticum', *Nature Genetics* 25 (2): 223–7.

Marshall, E. (2004) 'Patient advocate named co-inventor on patent for the PXE disease gene', *Science*, 305 (5668): 1226.

Novas, C. and Rose, N. (2000) 'Genetic risk and the birth of the somatic individual', *Economy and Society* 29 (4): 485–513.

PXE International (1996a) 'Blood and tissue registry', *PXE International Member-Gram* 1(2).

—— (1996b) 'PXE international awards its first biomedical grant to Jackson Laboratory', *PXE International MemberGram* 1 (3/4).

—— (1996c) 'Research', *PXE International MemberGram* 1(2).

—— (1998) 'Epidemiological study', *PXE International MemberGram* 3 (3/4).

—— (2005) 'PXE research 2004', *PXE International MemberGram* 10 (1): 5–24.

Rabeharisoa, V. (2003) 'The struggle against neuromuscular diseases in France and the emergence of the "partnership model" of patient organisation', *Social Science & Medicine*, 57 (11): 2127–36.

Rabeharisoa, V. and Callon, M. (2004) 'Patients and scientists in French muscular dystrophy research', in S. Jasanoff (ed.), *States of Knowledge: the co-production of science and social order*. London: Routledge.

Rabinow, P. (1996) *Essays on the Anthropology of Reason*. Princeton, NJ: Princeton University Press.

—— (1999) *French DNA: trouble in purgatory*. Chicago, IL: University of Chicago Press.

Rapp, R. (1999) *Testing Women, Testing the Fetus: the social impact of amniocentesis in America*. New York: Routledge.

—— (2003) 'Cell life and death, child life and death: genomic horizons, genetic diseases, family stories', in S. Franklin and M. M. Lock (eds), *Remaking Life and Death: toward an anthropology of the biosciences*. Oxford: James Currey.

Rapp, R., Taussig, K. S. and Heath, D. (2002) 'Genealogical disease: where hereditary abnormality, biomedical explanation, and family responsibility meet', in S. Franklin and S. McKinnon (eds), *Relative Matters: new directions in kinship study*. Durham, NC: Duke University Press.

Rose, N. and Novas, C. (2004) 'Biological citizenship', in A. Ong and S. Collier (eds), *Global Assemblages: technology, politics, and ethics as anthropological problems*. Malden, MA: Blackwell.

Shiva, V. (1997) *Biopiracy: the plunder of nature and knowledge*. Toronto: Between The Lines.

Shostak, S. (2004) 'Environmental justice and genomics: acting on the futures of environmental health', *Science as Culture*, 13 (4): 539–61.

Stockdale, A. (1999) 'Waiting for the cure: mapping the social relations of human gene therapy research', *Sociology of Health & Illness*, 21 (5): 579–96.

Stockdale, A. and Terry, S. F. (2002) 'Advocacy groups and the new genetics', in J. S. Alper, C. Ard, A. Asch, J. Beckwith, P. Conrad and L. N. Geller (eds), *The Double-Edged Helix: social implications of genetics in a diverse society*. Baltimore, MD: Johns Hopkins University Press.

Sunder Rajan, K. (2003) 'Genomic capital: public cultures and market logics of corporate biotechnology', *Science as Culture*, 12 (1): 87–121.

Terry, P. F. (2003a) 'PXE International: harnessing intellectual property law for benefit-sharing', in B. M. Knoppers (ed.), *Populations and Genetics: legal and socio-ethical perspectives*. Leiden: Martinus Nijhoff.

Terry, S. (1996) 'One person's perspective', *PXE International MemberGram* 1 (2).

—— (2003b) 'Benefit sharing for consumers'. Paper presented at Conference 'Toward an understanding of benefit sharing', Philadelphia, PA, 3 March.

—— (2003c) 'Learning genetics', *Health Affairs,* 22 (5): 166–70.

Terry, S. F. and Boyd, C. D. (2001) 'Researching the biology of PXE: partnering in the process', *American Journal of Medical Genetics,* 106: 177–84.

Terry, S. F. and Terry, P. F. (2001) 'A consumer perspective on informed consent and third-party issues', *Journal of Continuing Education in the Health Professions,* 21: 256–64.

Terry, S. F., Terry, P. F., Marais, A. S., Ronchetti, I. P., Le Roux, T., Boyd, C. D. and Bercovitch, L. (1999) 'The effect of one genetic support group on research for a rare disease'. Poster presented at the American Society of Human Genetics Annual Meeting, San Francisco, CA, 18–24 October.

Transgenomic (2002) 'Transgenomic signs collaboration agreement with lay advocacy group PXE International (Press Release)'. Available online at: http://www.pxe.org/research/transgenomic.html (accessed 14 August 2005).

van Soest, S., Swart, J., Tijmes, N., Sandkuijl, L. A., Rommers, J. and Bergen, A. A. (1997) 'A locus for autosomal recessive pseudoxanthoma elasticum, with penetrance of vascular symptoms in carriers, maps to chromosome 16p13.1', *Genome Research,* 7 (8): 830–4.

Waldby, C. (2000) *The Visible Human Project: informatic bodies and posthuman medicine.* London and New York: Routledge.

Yoxen, E. (1983) *The Gene Business: who should control biotechnology.* New York: Harper and Row.

Zavestoski, S., McCormick, S. and Brown, P. (2004) 'Gender, embodiment, and disease: environmental breast cancer activists' challenges to science, the biomedical model, and policy', *Science as Culture,* 13 (4): 563–86.

3 Patients as public in ethics debates
Interpreting the role of patients' organisations in democracy

Annemiek Nelis, Gerard de Vries and Rob Hagendijk

Introduction

In the past thirty years, patients' organisations have become major players in the healthcare system. Their sizes and shapes vary. Memberships vary from a few dozen to several thousand people. Many patients' organisations have professional staff – in some cases substantial ones – while others are run entirely by volunteers. Some patients' organisations are subsidised by pharmaceutical companies, others deliberately keep the industry at arm's length. Almost all patients' organisations have close links with the medical profession. Typically, physicians and medical experts serve on scientific advisory committees; occasionally they also sit on the board.

Established in the first place to serve practical purposes, patients' organisations enable people to meet others who suffer from the same or a similar disease and to share practical information and medical knowledge related to their condition. Occasionally patients' organisations also act as intermediaries between patients, care providers and insurance companies. Extending these primary, practical tasks, many patients' organisations have also become active in political arenas. They lobby politicians and the media to gain attention for their members and the problems they have to cope with. They comment on government policy proposals, partake in government advisory committees and represent the interests of patients at parliamentary hearings and other forums where government and the medical world meet. They thus offer a voice to people who – due to chronic disease or illness – have a limited opportunity to make themselves heard; patients' organisations are widely seen as welcome additions to the democratic process. They are perceived as encouraging what proponents of participatory democracy have called 'inclusion', i.e. the enrolment of people who traditionally have no or little voice in politics (Pateman 1970; Barber 1984; Young 1999).

Gradually, however, the political role of patients' organisations has expanded beyond representing the direct interests of individual patients and their relatives. Increasingly, patients' organisations contribute to debates on medical issues of a more general kind, including controversial medical ethical issues. For example, in recent years the Dutch umbrella organisation for parents' and patients' organisations of hereditary and congenital diseases (VSOP) has taken public stands on politically sensitive issues such as pre-symptomatic testing, the triple-test, pre-implantation diagnostics, medical research with patients incapable of giving informed consent, genetics and medical examination at work, neonatal screening for untreatable conditions, and patenting genetic material (VSOP 2004). Member organisations of the VSOP and other patients' organisations have also issued statements on contested subjects such as, for example, the use of embryonic stem cells in research. In other countries, patients' organisations have taken similar initiatives.

The role of patients' organisations in public disputes on ethical issues raises issues different from their role in matters that relate directly to the interests and practicalities of the people they represent. Illness strikes without regard to a person's ethical, political or religious views. We may therefore expect that in spite of sharing many interests, on ethically controversial issues the opinions of members of a patients' organisation may – and in fact often do – diverge. For example, whilst all patients will be interested in a cure for their disease, it is far from evident that they will all be ready to accept research that involves the use of embryos, even if that research comes with the promise of a future treatment for the illness. In cases where patients' organisations have contributed to ethical controversies such as the debates on embryonic stem cell research, the legitimacy of their role therefore deserves scrutiny.

In fact, discussions about legitimacy do not wait for social scientists and other analysts to enter the debate. In some cases, these debates emerge *within* a patients' organisation; in other cases, *outsiders* may question on whose behalf the organisation is taking a stand in an ethical debate, and why its views should be attributed weight.

In this chapter, we will argue that the legitimacy of public actions by patients' organisations also raises questions for *political theory*. An analysis of the role of patients' organisations in medical ethics debates may contribute to more general discussions about the role of public consultation in science and technology. In the past decade, public consultation has become a staple ingredient of innovation policy. For a long time, it had been widely assumed that adverse reactions towards new medical and technical developments resulted from ignorance and lack of knowledge amongst the general public, a situation, one would think, that could be resolved by providing more and better information. Over the past ten years, however, this view has declined. Since the early 1990s, a wide range of studies has shown that citizens *are* able to assess the consequences of science and technology for everyday concerns. It has been found that widespread public opposition results not primarily from lack of information, but rather from distrust of the authorities responsible for managing the widespread application of science and technology in practical affairs (EC-DGXII 1999; Hagendijk

2004). Moreover, changing relations of science and society have suggested the need for a new social 'contract' with science and for scientific knowledge that is 'socially robust' (Gibbons 1999; Nowotny *et al.* 2001). Policymakers have endorsed these ideas in their attempts to deal with public crises about issues like BSE, GM food and the anxieties about genetics (House of Lords 2000; CEC 2000, 2001). Rebuilding trust through participation has become a central issue in contemporary science policy. Consensus conferences, citizens' juries and government initiated public debates about controversial scientific and technological projects such as nuclear energy, recombinant DNA and genetically modified food, have been developed to help achieve this (Banthien *et al.* 2003). Patients' organisations, it has been argued, can also play an important role in these new forms of mediation (Callon 1999).

Notwithstanding the enthusiasm for the 'new modes of deliberation', the added value to democracy of the presence of patients' organisations in public consultations and decision-making about controversial ethical issues remains to be explored. To what extent can patients' organisations legitimately claim to represent patients on these issues? If a patients' organisation raises its voice about a controversial issue, what exactly does it achieve – in which respects does its contribution differ from other voices that are raised? Do patients' organisations add anything to the spectrum of opinions already expressed through other channels?

In this chapter, we will discuss the role of patients' organisations in ethically controversial issues related to scientific and technological developments. Interventions of Dutch and UK patients' organisations in debates on stem cell research for therapeutic cloning will serve as examples. Empirical details are based on written sources and on interviews with representatives of patients' organisations in the Netherlands and the UK conducted in 2003.

Stem cells are pluripotent, and it is claimed that they can develop into any tissue or organ. In therapeutic cloning, the stem cell's DNA is replaced by the DNA of another organism, the donor. Because cloned cells will be compatible with the donor's immune system, therapeutic cloning is claimed to be a promising route to therapies for a wide variety of disorders. Much-cited target diseases that are thought likely to benefit in the near future from stem cell research are Parkinson's disease, Alzheimer's disease and diabetes. Although it is also possible to use adult stem cells, which can be found in bone marrow, for therapeutic cloning, scientists claim there is irrefutable technical justification for favouring embryonic stem cells. These cells are harvested from what are called 'excess embryos' that originate from IVF treatment cycles, or they are specifically grown for the purpose of stem cell research. These procedures have however become the subject of fierce controversy in several countries. Since the 1990s, the debates have focused on one question in particular: is it legitimate to use embryos for therapeutic cloning, that is, to use stem cells from embryos for the creation of tissue or organs? To many, and in particular to various Christian churches, the use of excess embryos and embryos that have been created for the instrumental purpose of stem cell research is a clear violation of respect for human life and for that reason should be completely proscribed. Non-religious groups have also opposed the use of embryos for therapeutic cloning, among other things because of fears that it will lead to a commercialization of human life. Debates about this issue have led to different forms of national regulation. Whilst Germany legally bans all research in the use of embryos, the United States allows private enterprise to undertake embryo research but forbids public institutions to do so (Gottweis 2002). In the United Kingdom the law allows researchers to use embryos for research up to fourteen days after fertilization. In the Netherlands, the use of embryos for stem cell research is allowed, but under stricter conditions than those which apply in the UK.

'We have accountability in place'

Given the diversity of ethical views and standpoints, a patients' organisation's public support for a controversial issue such as stem cell research raises questions about legitimacy. This is not just a matter of theoretical interest. In fact, patients' organisations often have to address these questions in their internal discussions, or are invited to do so by critical outsiders.

Internal discussions may be initiated for several reasons. Despite the promissory claims that stem cell research holds for Parkinson's and Alzheimer's disease and for diabetes, in the UK only the Parkinson Disease Society (PDS) has taken an explicit stand both in the media and in parliamentary debates on this subject. The organisations representing sufferers of Alzheimer's disease and diabetes patients did not publicly address stem cell research. Questioned about this difference in one of our interviews, the PDS staff explained that Diabetes UK did not take a public position on stem cell research because its board of trustees was internally divided on the issue. The reason the Alzheimer's Society had refrained from taking a public stand was different, according to the PDS staff. Following the publication of an opinion on living wills, the Alzheimer's Society had been targeted by 'pro-life' groups and had met a lot of hostile press. As a result, the society had experienced a major drop in donations. When faced again with the question whether it should publicly address another controversial issue, this time stem cell research, the society concluded that it could not afford to do so.

Critical outsiders may also question the legitimacy of a patients' organisation's public statements on ethically controversial issues. For example, in a hearing on stem cell research organised by the UK parliament, a conservative MP explicitly asked the PDS's Head of Policy, Research and Information whether the views he had put forward were his own opinions or the views of his members. Reflecting on the event, the director emphasised that the opinions he had expressed were clearly those of PDS members. 'We have accountability in place,' he declared (interview, 8 May 2003).

When invited to elaborate on this, the PDS director explained that, before formulating its statement, the board of the PDS had first informed itself thoroughly about the issue of stem cell research. To that end, it had sought support from its scientific advisory board. The scientific advisory board turned out to be unanimously in favour of stem cell research. Moreover, he pointed out, the Royal Society, the Medical Research Council, the Association of Medical Research Charities, as well as several individual researchers and research institutes, had expressed similar views. In June 2000, the UK's Chief Medical Officer had also favourably reported on stem cell research for medical treatment opportunities. However, emphasised the PDS director, his organisation had not only consulted experts but also the members of the society. At a PDS annual meeting that took place two months after the publication of the Chief Medical Officer's report on stem cell research, members of the PDS had been asked to identify the top three issues the society should take forward in its campaigns. The majority of PDS members attending the annual meeting had put stem cell research at the top of their list. The conservative MP's question whether the PDS represented the standpoint of its members could therefore be answered affirmatively, according to the PDS director. The PDS had legitimately claimed to represent the views of its members. With 28,000 members and the support of all major medical authorities, added the director, 'we have enough weight and critical mass to have prominence'.

An interview with the director of the Dutch Parkinson's patients' society (PPV) – an organisation with about 7,000 members and a professional staff of eight part-time employees – showed a different line of reasoning. When it came to stem cell research, according to its director, the PPV did not so much *represent* its members; rather, it had *informed* them.

In the spring of 2003, the PPV board had prepared a policy document suggesting that the time had come for the PPV publicly to address a number of controversial issues, including stem cell research. When interviewed, the PPV director emphasised that, whilst the majority of the members present at the subsequent annual meeting had eventually supported the policy, the idea that the PPV as a whole had taken a stand on stem cell research required to be nuanced. Stem cell research is not something that many people know much about, he stressed. Although PPV members in general are very positive about new scientific developments, he said, 'they really have no idea what this is about' (interview with Nelis, 1 April 2003). In contrast to the PPV board, which has close links with the scientific community through its scientific advisory board and thus had the opportunity to inform itself thoroughly, ordinary PPV members had little opportunity to become really acquainted with the details of the issue, explained the PPV director. He therefore perceived his society as having the task of informing its members about stem cell research and about what, in the interest of their own lives and that of future generations, PPV members *should* think about stem cell research. In line with this policy, the PPV subsequently invited the neurosurgeon Dr J. Staal to give a talk on the 'facts and fictions of stem cell research' at the PPV annual meeting in November 2003. At the end of his talk, Dr Staal asked the audience to fill in a questionnaire to indicate what they thought about stem cell research. According to the minutes of the meeting, the majority of the members present at the meeting were in favour of stem cell research and saw no ethical objections to it. They also thought that decisions about this type of research 'should be a matter of the patients involved and not a matter of politics' (PPV 2003).

The self-assuredness with which the UK patients' organisation presented its statements as representing the views of its members seems to contrast sharply with the Dutch PPV, whose director had a much more cautious interpretation of this issue. The PPV director, however, showed a different kind of self-assuredness, in that he believes himself to be in a position to tell his members what they should think – thus opening the possibility of being charged with paternalism. In spite of these differences, however, the efforts that both organizations had put into preparing and backing up their public statements are strikingly similar. In both cases, scientific articles were consulted to learn more about stem cell research and its promises, and advice had been sought from experts closely involved in stem cell research. In both cases, some of these experts were members of the scientific advisory board of the patients' organisation. When the boards had made up their minds, both the PDS and the PPV consulted their members in a rather informal way, i.e. by asking members attending the organisation's annual meeting to deliver their opinion about stem cell research, either by rating (PDS) or by filling in a questionnaire (PPV). In both cases, the consultation took place almost immediately after members had been explicitly informed about the promises of stem cell research – in the UK case by a widely publicised and positively-toned government report; in the Dutch case after an oral presentation of the promises of stem cell research by a leading Dutch expert in the field. Discussions had taken place mainly within the board and between the board and scientific advisory commissions. However, in both cases one may question whether the organisations had actively tried to inform their members about alternative views and about arguments that oppose stem cell research. No traces of such views were to be found, either on the organisations' websites or in their magazines.

In spite of their remarkably similar course, the interpretation the directors gave to legitimise their actions diverged. It seems fair to say that, if the PDS director can claim to represent the members of his organization, the PPV can do the same; and if the activities of the PPV director are open for a paternalism charge, the same holds for his PDS counterpart. The problem that we run into is, however, not in the perceptions of the two directors; rather, it is bound up with an ambiguity in the concept of political 'representation'.

Representation in politics

In a study on the history of the concept of 'representation' and its role in political thought, Hanna Fenichel Pitkin has distinguished two major meanings of the term (Pitkin 1989). Both meanings result from what Pitkin presents as the inherent paradox of representation: 'making present in *some* sense what is nevertheless *not* literally present' (Pitkin 1989: 142). As a result of this paradox there are two opposing answers to the question of what someone elected as a representative is supposed to do: he can either express what those he represents prefer or think, or, once elected, he can defend what he himself thinks is rational or right. The discrepancy between the two meanings of 'representation' has become associated with numerous issues in political theory, Pitkin shows, such as questions about the role of political parties, referenda, citizens' initiatives and the relationship between local issues and national politics.

The difference between the two meanings becomes manifest, for example, in parliamentary democracies with constituency voting systems. Does an MP in such a system speak on behalf of the voters of his own constituency, or is he, once elected by his home constituency, a member of a parliament which – in the much-cited words of Edmund Burke – 'is not a congress of ambassadors from different and hostile interests ... but ... a deliberative assembly of one nation, with one interest, that of the whole'? (Burke 1949). If we adopt the first meaning of representation, we may expect MPs frequently to consult the citizens of the district which voted them into parliament and to defend the interests of those districts. If we go along with the second meaning of the term, there is neither a duty to follow the preferences of voters, nor an *a priori* reason to let the interests of the district prevail. The interest of the nation – the public good – is supposed to have significance of its own and not to coincide with the aggregate of individual viewpoints and desires. Burke told the electors of Bristol:

> If the local constituent should have an interest, or should form a hasty opinion, evidently opposite to the real good of the rest of the community, the Member for that place ought to be as far as any other from any endeavour to give it effect.

Parallel to the theoretical difference between the two meanings of representation, there is an obvious, practical, down-to-earth difference between views of what Members of Parliament are supposed to do to become a legitimate spokesperson. In the first view, MPs need first and foremost to maintain contact with their constituency, and they will have to consult them regularly in order to learn their opinions on specific subjects. In the second view, however, MPs should first of all inform themselves about an issue in order to develop a well founded, balanced idea about the public good that is at stake. Especially when issues that also involve technical questions are discussed, we may expect an MP who adopts the second view to visit a library or to consult experts, rather than to meet his constituency in the back room of a local pub to hear their uninformed opinions.

In practice, of course, most MPs will attempt to balance both views, and this holds for patients' organisations too. Where representatives of patients' organisations explicitly present themselves as spokespersons for the direct interests of patients – for example in matters related to the care or to the practicalities of life of people with an illness or disability – they tend to speak in the name of their members and put forward and defend the interest of those members. The legitimacy of their views is based on frequent consultations with members about their interests and needs. However, where patients' organisations contribute to debates on controversial ethical issues such as stem cell research, the situation is more complicated. The Dutch PPV director may be said to have adopted Burke's second position. His organisation did not claim to represent what his members thought, but rather it set out what it conceived as the proper view on stem cell research. On Burke's interpretation of 'representation', the director could rightly have claimed that this is what he, as an elected representative, is supposed to do. In contrast, the UK PDS director clearly favoured the first meaning of 'representation', as distinguished by Pitkin. However, as we observed above, the consent of PDS members was invited only after the PDS board had convinced itself that a public statement in favour of stem cell research was called for. In spite of the emphasis the PDS director put on the event, consultation of PDS members was organised in a rather informal way.

To make up their minds about an issue that is supposed to relate to the 'public good' but that is deeply technical and still full of uncertainties in the way that stem cell research is, both the British and the Dutch Parkinson patients' organisations relied on experts they perceived to be authorities on the issue. Their scientific advisory boards served as mediators to set up links with those experts. Although in ethical matters there is a wide range of other authoritative institutions available (for example the churches, as well as non-religious organisations), both patients' organisations chose to exclusively consult the medical and scientific world.

Following this course of action, the patients' organisations are however in danger of ending up in a situation in which the legitimacy of their views on ethical issues depends exclusively on their concurrence with views supported by the medical establishment. If this is the case, what is the added value of the patients' organisations' contributions to the debate? Are they simply repeating what their scientific advisors say? Or, expressed more cynically, is the contribution of patients' organisations to the public debate perhaps only to add 'spin' to the views of the medical establishment, i.e. of the money-hungry research community and the pharmaceutical industry?

Perceived from both of the views on representation that Pitkin distinguishes, the contribution of patients' organisations to debates about controversial ethical issues seems to be limited indeed. Duplicating arguments that have already been put forward forcefully by others, i.e. those in the medical world, patients' organisations seem vulnerable to the accusation that they add little more than 'spin' to the views of parties that have little trouble making themselves heard in modern societies. In the latter view, patients may represent the views of their constituency, if these views do not differ from those brought forward by others; it is questionable what their added value is in democratic debate. However, when we look at patients' organisations not as presenting (other people's) arguments and ideas but as presenting *proof* for arguments and ideas, we may start to see their contribution in a different light.

To back up this claim, a detour to political theory is necessary. An argument proposed by the American philosopher John Dewey may help us reach a more appropriate view of the role of patients' organisations.

The presence of a public

After an absence of several decades, Dewey's name re-entered mainstream philosophical discussions during the 1970s. Among political scientists, however, his work is still hardly known. Recent textbooks on democracy, for example Held (1996) and Dahl *et al.* (2003), do not mention Dewey's views on politics, nor does Kymlicka's (2002) well-known textbook on political philosophy. The unfamiliarity with Dewey's work may be caused by his unusual conceptualisation of politics. While the pluralist, participation and deliberative views of democracy fit seamlessly with common-sense ideas, Dewey chose to take a contra-intuitive, albeit in his view more realistic, starting point to analyse what politics is about.

Mainstream views perceive democracy as a specific way to organise the political process, i.e. as a set of procedures for a given community to decide collectively about a common (e.g. national) course of action. In this view, 'state' and 'politics' are closely connected terms – the democratic political process prepares for state rule – and questions about legitimacy centre around the relation between rulers and ruled. Democracy, in this view, is simply government for and by the people. In a democracy, the legitimacy of the actions of rulers is based on their being the representatives of the ruled.

Dewey takes another tack. According to Dewey, politics is not primarily a matter of a community of people negotiating and discussing their opinions, views and interests to decide upon a common course of action. For Dewey, politics emerges in situations where people are strangers to each other but nevertheless have to cope with the consequences of each other's transactions. If that happens, a *public* comes into being, consisting of 'all those who are affected by the indirect consequences of transactions to such an extent that it is deemed necessary to have those consequences systematically cared for' (Dewey 1927: 15–16). As different private transactions will have consequences for different groups of people not involved in those actions, the term 'public' is a relative one. Moreover, there is no *a priori* reason to assume that those who are part of a public are socially related to, or even know, one another. A 'public' is clearly a different kind of entity than a 'community'. The community that the standard view supposes as given may be a *result* of political action, but it is not the point of departure of the analysis.

A public needs to be organised and, according to Dewey, this is the primary function of the state. 'The state is the organisation of the public effected through officials for the protection of the interests shared by its members' (Dewey 1927: 33). A democratic state distinguishes itself among other things by its *effects*: attention and respect for everyone who is part of a public; tolerance for and protection of minorities; and equality before the law. In the words of Dewey's biographer Ryan, Dewey thought that democracy should 'be committed to re-creating in an industrial society (i.e. a society of strangers) the mutual comprehension and appreciation that we experience in "face-to-face" communities' (Ryan 1995: 219).

Dewey's vision does not lead to radically different answers to the question of how a democratic state should be organised. Rule of law, free elections and a free press, for example, are also key institutional arrangements in Dewey's view on democracy. The role of these institutions, however, differs in Dewey's interpretation from the one implied in mainstream democratic theory. They are appreciated for their effects. On this reading, for example, a free press is not a channel to air the voices of community members, but an instrument to bring public causes into the open (cf. also De Vries 2002, 2003).

Apart from the state, other organisations may also help to organise a public. Patients' organisations may be interpreted as contributing to that task. They help to make visible which (potential) indirect consequences of private actions emerge for patients, thus making clear that a specific public is at stake.

Under a Deweyan interpretation, the business of patients' organisations is not to *represent* patients but to *present* patients *as a public* that needs support, attention and care. Individual patients who may or may not have much in common thus become a public with a name and a face; an address. Patients thus become a referent in a public debate. The public that is at stake becomes a political *fact*. This has an important consequence. When the legitimacy of the actions of the patients' organisation is questioned, the key question to be raised to a patients' organisation is no longer 'can you convincingly show that you represent the views of the community of patients?', but 'can you convincingly prove that there is a public that has to be taken care of, i.e. that your concerns have a referent?'

These two questions point in different directions. As suggested by the conventional view of politics, the first invites a patients' organisation to show that there is a *similarity* between the views it publicises and those of its members. This, however, leads to the problems we have set out before. In the case of controversial medical ethical issues about innovative technologies bound up with complicated technical questions and uncertainties such as stem cell research, it is hard to know what one's members want (and questionable whether members themselves *do* or *can* know what they want). As we have shown, organisations will have to resort either to paternalism, i.e. to present views that they *suppose* their members will have once they have been exposed to the right kind of arguments, or to representation, e.g. to claim the constituency has been *asked* what it is it 'really wants'. Moreover, following this line of reasoning, patients' organisations are vulnerable to the accusation that they are only parroting the views of the medical establishment. In contrast, the second Deweyan question invites the patients' organisation to *document the steps that link the issue to the patients* that it claims are involved as a public. The organisation has convincingly to show that patients are a public in the debate about a controversial research procedure, e.g. stem cell research. The patients' organisation has to present the *referent* of the debate.

Bringing it home: the presentation of proof

If the role of patients' organisations in political debate is to prove there is a public at stake that needs to be taken care of, what exactly do patients' organisations need to *do* to fulfil this role? They have to present the patient as a public, in the same way an experimental scientist has to present his results to back up an hypothesis. An obvious way to achieve this is literally to introduce patients in a debate. Showing the disease or the impact of a disease on a real person's life is like showing experimental evidence: *this* is what we are talking about; these are the people who as a public need to be taken care of.

Professional spokespersons of patients' organisations invited to represent patients at hearings or at press conferences indeed often choose to be accompanied by one or two patients. As the PDS staff explained in an interview:

> [I]t is important to involve people with conditions, because it is all very well speaking about the benefits of science or talking about the rights of embryos of four days or five days old, but to meet people with Parkinson's disease is a different matter. There is one woman ... 44 years of age and with Parkinson's, who has been very active and who has repeatedly taken a public stand in stem cell debates. To speak to her about her hopes and her fears brings it home to people: this is actually what we are talking about.
>
> (Interview, 8 May 2003)

Introduced to the room where a debate about stem cell research is taking place, the 44-year-old patient makes Parkinson's patients present as a public in those debates. On the spot, she provides a referent to the discussions about stem cell research: 'It is *me* you are talking about.' She does not just 'illustrate' or support the claims that are made by the patients' organisations, she actually proves there is a public waiting for a cure or treatment to release them from their suffering.

Presenting patients as 'proof' of the claim that there is a public that needs to be taken care of may be compared with the presentation of experimental proof within the natural sciences. However, as every scientist who has ever performed an experiment knows, to present experimental proof, i.e. to add reality to a claim, requires *work*: preparation, organisation and instruments. While science is traditionally portrayed as the endeavour to mimic or represent nature, many scholars today accept that scientific work does not represent nature itself but actively shapes and creates what we tend to call 'nature'. 'Hard facts' are the result of hard work. It requires a lot of effort to set up an undisputable chain of links between the statements published in a scientific paper and the phenomena the paper claims to describe and explain.

The task facing someone who wants to operate in a political arena involves similar efforts. Patients' organisations can provide the means to achieving this aim. Having close contacts with their members, patients' organisations may invite patients who are particularly talented in presenting their cause to attend important meetings, hearings and press-conferences. The 44-year-old patient referred to by the PDS staff in our interview has presented her case 'again and again' in stem cell debates. Patients as public are not 'naturally' given, but are the result of work. To effectively present herself as the public in a debate, the patient has to be properly introduced, and may even have been instructed and trained. Experimental scientists have to prepare their materials and fine-tune their instruments to make a convincing case; likewise, patients' organisations have to put a lot of effort and organisation to present their constituency as a public.

The difference between 'talking in the name of' a public and 'presenting' a public rests in the actual confrontation of the audience with this public (e.g. with patients). When Austin Smith, director of the Institute for Stem Cell Research in Edinburgh, addressed the Members of the European Parliament who had to take a vote on a proposal to ban stem cell research, he told the MEPs to ask themselves whether they can deny patients the prospect of developing a cure in favour of an entity that contains no heart, blood or nerve cells and is destined only to be destroyed or to be kept frozen forever.

They have got to be able to stand in front of someone with Parkinson's disease and say I don't care about you – all I care about is this little ball of cells. And they should be prepared to justify their position to the people of Europe.

(Smith 2003)

Bringing patients to public hearings, public meetings and public debates, patients' organisations turn the hypothetical situation that Smith suggests into reality. In a similar vein, pro-life organisations present a different public: the unborn foetus (described by Austin as a mere ball of cells) with a right to life. Using pictures and images of unborn foetuses, pro-life organisations make a similar claim to that of patients' organisations: 'this is the public that needs to be looked after'.

The actions of the American movie star Michael J. Fox may serve as an extreme illustration of how a public is made present in political debate. Fox, who has juvenile Parkinson's disease, appeared in September 1999 at a US Appropriations Subcommittee Hearing to petition for federal funding for research into Parkinson's disease. In his autobiography, Fox explains how he prepared for the event:

> I made a deliberate choice to appear before the subcommittee without medication. It seemed to me that this occasion demanded that my testimony about the effect of the disease, and the urgency we as a community were feeling, be *seen* as well as heard. For people who had never observed me in this kind of shape, the transformation must have been startling.
>
> (Fox 2002: 296–7)

Invoking a *technique* to show the severity of his symptoms, i.e. by deliberately abstaining from his usual medication, Fox's plea for federal research funding for Parkinson's was coupled with his producing a referent.

As in the case of scientific experiments, in which a single experiment is used to illustrate something that is claimed to be true irrespective of time and place, Fox is not just presenting his own case. He is presenting himself as an exemplar of a much larger group of patients. In this sense, he really presents a *public* in its broadest sense.

> I am not here because I am in trouble. Or rather I *am* – along with nearly one and a half million other Parkinson's patients on whose behalf I appear – *in serious trouble,* but of a kind far graver than any group of senators could ever cause.
>
> (Fox 2002: 294)

Of course, researchers and clinicians may make similar claims for research money by arguing *in the name of* their patients. However, the gap between debating *about* patients and having a debate *with* a patient is as great as the difference between a hypothesis and the outcome of an experiment.

When convincingly confronted with the existence of a referent, a political fact emerges that is hard to neglect. Fox proves his point: people like him are the public we are talking about.

Conclusions

In the recent past, it has often been argued that techno-scientific societies are in need of new approaches to organise democracy. Political scientists and Science and Technology Studies (STS) scholars, amongst others, have made suggestions for new forms of deliberation – in particular between experts and lay people – to achieve this new democratic thinking. With a few exceptions, these suggestions aim at extending the number of participants to be included in political debates. Patients' organisations are widely welcomed as a way to achieve this goal.

The common view of the role of patients' organisations, however, cannot account for the contributions of patients' organisations to current debates on issues in medical ethics about technologies that are still bound up with many uncertainties and technical questions. As we have seen in the case of the two Parkinson societies, the UK PDS and the Dutch PPV, patients' organisations necessarily depend on the view of (medical) experts, while in their approach to their own members they may either organise their role in representing the views of their constituency, or act as informer and educator of their constituency. Both approaches run the risk of being perceived as parroting the medical authorities. When patients' organisations are invited to defend the legitimacy of their interventions, the range of possible answers is limited and ultimately unconvincing.

The Deweyan perspective on politics that we have defended in this chapter allocates patients' organisations a different role. Rather than *representing* patients, they *present* patients as a public in medical ethical debates. We have argued that Dewey's perspective enables us to appreciate the contribution of patients because it clarifies how and why patients' organisations help to bring patients into the debate, and thus provide the debate with a referent that has a name and an address. In this sense, patients bring something to the debate that others (in particular medical experts) are not able to provide: the presentation of (often confrontation with) the public that needs to be looked after. The unique thing that patients and their organisations can do is to make themselves present in the debate as *the public* concerned. Others may represent them or mobilise them as such, but they can do so only in the role of supporting actor, ambassador or spokesperson. Their legitimacy is and should always be open to question.

Patients' organisations may use a variety of techniques to perform this function and it is therefore precisely on this point that their role stands out from that of the medical establishment. This does not, of course, reduce the danger of medical authorities mobilising patients' organisations for their own arguments and their own interests. But it does mean, however, that patients' organisations may re-think their position in ethical debates about technologies which are bound up with uncertainties.

References

Banthien, H., Jaspers, M. and Renner, A. (2003) 'Governance of the European research area: the role of civil society', Final Report. Bensheim: IFOK.

Barber, B. (1984) *Strong Democracy*. Berkeley, CA: Berkeley University Press.

Burke, E. (1949) 'Speech to the Electors of Bristol', in Ross J. S. Hoffman and Paul Levack (eds), *Burke's Politics*. New York: Alfred A. Knopf. Available online at http://press-pubs.uchicago.edu/founders/documents/v1ch13s7.html (accessed 11 July 2006).

Callon, M. (1999) 'The role of lay people in the production and dissemination of scientific knowledge', *Science, Technology and Society*, 4 (1): 81–94.

Commission of the European Communities (CEC) (2000) *Science, Society and the Citizen in Europe*. Brussels: European Commission.

—— (2001) *European Governance: a white paper*. Brussels: CEC.

Dahl, R. A., Shapiro, I. and Chebub, J. A. (eds) (2003) *The Democracy Source Book*. Cambridge, MA: MIT Press.

Dewey, J. (1927) *The Public and Its Problems*. Athens, OH: Swallow Press – Ohio University Press.

EC-DGXII (1999) *The Europeans and Modern Biotechnology. Eurobarometer 46.1* (Brussels: EC-DGXII, 1997).

Fox, M. J. (2002) *Lucky Man. A Memoir*. New York: Hyperion Press.

Gibbons, M. (1999) 'Science's New Contract with Society', *Nature*, 402, 2 (Supplement, 1999), C81–4.

Gottweis, H. (2002) 'Stem cell policies in the United States and in Germany: between bioethics and regulation', *Policy Studies Journal*, 30(4): 444–69.

Hagendijk, R. P. (2004) 'The public understanding of science and public participation in regulated worlds', *Minerva*, 42: 41–59.

Held, D. (1996) *Models of Democracy*. Oxford: Polity Press.

House of Lords Select Committee on Science and Technology (2000) *Science and Society*. London: The Stationery Office.

Kymlicka, W. (2002) *Contemporary Political Philosophy*. Oxford: Oxford University Press.

Nowotny, H., Scott, P. and Gibbons, M. (2001) *Rethinking Science: knowledge and the public in an age of uncertainty*. London: Polity Press.

Pateman, C. (1970) *Participation and Democratic Theory*. Cambridge: Cambridge University Press.

Pitkin, H. F. (1989) 'Representation', in T. Ball, J. Farr and R. S. Hanson (eds) *Political Innovation and Conceptual Change*. Cambridge: Cambridge University Press.

PPV (2003) 'Feiten en Ficties van Stamcelonderzoek'. Available online at http://www.parkinson-vereniging.nl/pages/stamcellen feiten en fictie.html (accessed 19 July 2006).

Ryan, A. (1995) *John Dewey and the High Tide of American Liberalism*. New York: W.W. Norton.

Smith, A. (2003) 'Why I believe Brussels must not outlaw stem cell research'. Available online at http://www.iscr.ed.ac.uk/news/press-releases-2003apr17.html (accessed 11 July 2006).

Vries, G. H. de (2002) 'Doen we het zo goed? De plaats van het publieke debat over medische ethiek in een democratie', *Krisis. Tijdschrift voor Filosofie*, 4: 39–59.

—— (2003) 'Democratie, pragmatisme en publieke debatten over medische ethiek', in I. Devisch and G. Verschraegen (eds), *De Verleiding van de Ethiek. Over de plaats van morele argumenten in de huidige maatschappij*. Amsterdam: Boom.

VSOP (2004) 'Dossiers en standpunten'. Available online at http://www.vsop.nl/dossiers/index.php (accessed 10 July 2006).

Young, I. M. (1999) 'Justice, inclusion and deliberative democracy', in S. Macedo (ed.), *Deliberative Politics: essays on democracy and disagreement*. Oxford: Oxford University Press.

4 From 'scraps and fragments' to 'whole organisms'

Molecular biology, clinical research and post-genomic bodies

Susan E. Kelly

Introduction

The general classification 'post-genomics' encompasses a broad array of topic areas and approaches associated with generating higher biological meaning and function out of raw sequence data. The multiple approaches now engaged by the increasingly heterogeneous and overlapping socio-technical networks of post-genomic research are envisioned to converge in systems-level models of human and other biological organisms. With accelerating knowledge of molecular biology, biochemical and physiological pathways, it now appears possible to envision systems understanding of the human organism grounded at the molecular level (Hunter 2003; Kitano 2002). According to Geoffrey Duyk in a recent *Nature Genetics* article:

> The key challenge for the coming century will be to establish complete molecular descriptions of biological processes that are sufficiently quantitative and dynamic to allow their predictive modeling or simulation. Parallel development of enhanced data visualization tools, in addition to the ongoing challenges of data storage, computation and analysis will be increasingly central to these endeavors. In the end, we would like to be able to map gene activity onto physiological processes.
>
> (Duyk 2002: 465)

My aim in this chapter is to explore a framework for an emerging ethics of post-genomic science that is centred in the material and metaphorical production of bodies. This focus – drawing on social studies of technoscience – provides insight into normative structures of social relations embedded within scientific and technological 'visions' that are an integral part of the social shaping of technology (e.g. Brown *et al.* 2000). Recent scholarship examining the cultural and material production of bodies associated with technoscience suggests that the activities and interests of groups involved in innovation processes are encoded within their particular boundaries and in the production of new individual and collective identities (Clarke *et al.*

2003; Downey and Dumit 1997; Lock, Young and Cambrosio 2000; Haraway 1997).

I suggest that movement in the life sciences, from the 'scraps and fragments' (Haldane, quoted in Ausiello 2000) of genes, proteins and cells, to the complexity of whole organisms, will entail not only new understandings of health and disease, but new production of bodies – a post-genomic body. The current metaphor of the 'genetic body' may be instructive in terms of the processes of its production, its relationships to biomedical research and clinical practices, and its manifestation in subjectivities and forms of governmentality (Bunton and Petersen 2005). In this chapter I will explore the production and constitution of post-genomic bodies as the site of conceptual reconstruction, technological innovation and identity production at the centre of emerging post-genomic sciences. I emphasise the production of metaphorical and material bodies through the visions and articulations of post-genomic scientific activities as sites of emerging ethics – both ethics as it has become manifest as a widely accepted conceptual framework for identifying and debating social implications of technology, and ethics as an expression of normative social relations that emerge at the productive interfaces of science, technology and society. I will argue that examination of visions of post-genomic science suggests shifting locations of risk, responsibility and accountability for which current ethical frameworks may be inadequate.

The recently published road map, or vision statement, of the US National Human Genome Research Institute (NHGRI) (Collins *et al.* 2003) is evidence that federally funded and industry scientists share an interest in capitalising on the successes of genome sequencing to produce tangible and significant improvements in health technologies. Research relationships are being transformed by the reliance of researchers across academia and industry on massive databases and other collaborative resources. Computational methods are becoming central to biological research to manage the amount and complexity of data emerging about the structure, function and dynamics of genes, proteins, cells, pathways, disease processes and broader phenotypic levels. Standardisation and integration of computational elements and processes will be of increasing significance, both in the integration of data into systems models, and in the simulation of complex, system-level interactions. Post-genomic science is envisioned to radically evolve disease concepts and disease nosologies in ways that will likely impact upon clinical practice and social experiences of illness at least as profoundly as has human genetics to date.

Like systems themselves, the production of systems-level biological knowledge is emergent and dynamic, and involves the integration of multiple and previously unconnected disciplines, the development of new disciplines, and significant technological innovation (Bruun 2006). To its proponents, the achievement of systems understanding of the human organism is viewed as the main development of the biological sciences in this century.

Ethics – ethical, social and legal implications or ELSI analysis – as represented in the NHGRI roadmap is an institutionalised knowledge-producing endeavour operating within constraints of intellectual community, expertise, discourse and practice (Kelly 2003). Within its vision of post-genomics, the roadmap suggests reconfiguring ethics activities into another branch of genomics or, at least, one of the tools of its translation into application, an instrumentality (Rothman 1994). Concepts including 'big ELSI', 'translational ELSI' and ELSI data-base tools 'analogous to the publicly accessible genomic maps and sequence databases that have accelerated other genomics research' (Collins *et al.* 2003: 845) suggest ethical analysis modelled on post-genomic science itself. Ethics analysis, in this sense, has become something of a 'human technique' (Ellul 1964), a form of social organisation adapting the human to the requirements of technology. An alternative perspective, drawn from studies of technoscience, suggests attention to ethics as normative social relations, identities and governmentalities emerging from and embedded within the production of new scientific knowledge and technologies (cf. Kelly 2006). Emerging ethics is inflected, but not subsumed, by 'the addition of a context of *implication* to the traditional context of application' (Glasner 2002), indicating that science and science production are increasingly sensitive to social impacts and public perceptions.

My analysis of post-genomics and ethics draws from visions of post-genomic science as represented in academic and industry literatures. I draw also from what are at present preliminary observations from a recently initiated case-based study of science and scientists engaged in the application of post-genomic tools and knowledges to experimental clinical practice. The purpose of the study is to examine potential changes in disease concepts, the social relations of knowledge production including the clinical and experimental enrolment of patients as human subjects, and the motivating visions or expectations of technologies, commodities and practices. It involves in-depth, sequential interviews with life scientists and clinicians involved in molecular biological research and associated with the interdisciplinary research programmes in molecular targets and translational research related to cancer. The research case studies being developed include a research programme to identify genetic and molecular predisposition markers for sporadic upper gastrointestinal cancer, and the clinical trials process of an experimental drug designed to intervene at a novel molecular site on solid-tumour cancer cells.

The genetic body

The Human Genome Project (HGP) has profoundly affected the types of explanation given within medicine, and in society more broadly, for a range of human diseases, characteristics and behaviours. The 'genetic body' (Turney and Balmer 1998, cited in Martin 1999) is a productive metaphor

that has emerged from recent analyses of these changes to capture transformations, not only in disease concepts, but in the modes of production,
technoscientific identities, social relations, and broader interfaces with
biomedical, cultural and governmental modalities that have characterised
the genetic era. The genetic body is in part constituted by emphasis on
genes as both the building blocks of life and the locus of disease aetiology.
Within this conceptual framework, the genetic endowment we inherit ultimately determines our health status, even while environmental and social
factors may play a role in the onset of disease. A relatively small set of rare
inherited conditions have been identified that are 'caused' by single faulty
genes, while more common diseases such as heart disease and diabetes are
believed to have a significant genetic component. The reduction of disease
causality to genes has been expanded to a range of behavioural disorders
or characteristics including schizophrenia, depression, alcoholism and
novelty-seeking, furthering the encroachment of genetic explanations on
identities and subjectivities.

The clinical application of genetic testing and screening to a number of
diseases, including familial breast and colon cancers, Huntington's disease,
Tay Sachs disease and cystic fibrosis, has given rise to a new language
of risk and new illness identities. Individuals may now be acutely, and
often inaccurately, aware of 'being at risk', experiencing 'mutation anxiety'
and 'presymptomatic disease', and being motivated to act by genetic
responsibility (Hallowell 1999; Parsons and Atkinson 1992; Cox and
McKellin 1999). Genetic risk concepts are engaged subjectively, becoming
elements of identity as well as illness experience. Bearing a disease mutation, being identified as 'at genetic risk' for disease, or exercising autonomy
by refusing such information, are emerging as expressions of embodiment
and relationship to disease. As such, they may form the basis of collective groupings, biosocial identities and biosocialities (Rabinow 1992) as
well as societal divisions. Through the possibility of routine genetic intervention into human reproduction, private reproductive decisions have
become entangled with public discourses and identities related to disability
and abortion (Parens and Asch 1999; Lippman 1991). Shared experiences
of risk, fate and location within systems of medical specialists, genetic
counsellors and other forms of narrative production are significant to
the constitution of genetic bodies. These experiences, and their manifestation in decision-making, illness behaviour and kinship relations, have
formed a significant element of the social and ethical analysis of the new
genetics.

In this context, it is genetic information itself, and its social consequences of potential employment and insurance discrimination, psycho-
social and kinship impacts, that have emerged as central forms of genetic
risk. Further, the separation of disease aetiology into genetic or environmental causes has bifurcated the location of responsibility (and agency) for
health. While positing 'genes' as the predominant sites of biomedical

research and explanatory activity, geneticisation of bodies has been accompanied by the rise of preventive medicine, lifestyle surveillance and individual responsibility for health (Clarke *et al.* 2003; Nelkin and Andrews 1999).

The metaphor of the genetic body thus captures important interplay among technological innovation, technoscientific visions, the organisation of medical practice, ethical and social implications analysis, and illness identities. Most powerfully, this has entailed writing the human directly into the genetic code, privileging single gene action over forms of complexity, and identifying 'risk' without concurrent ability to treat. The genetic body, the cultural product of the new genetics, is predicated upon the 'shared misunderstanding' of the relationship between genes and disease (Latour, quoted in Rheinberger 2000: 20).

Post-genomic biomedical research is anticipated to encompass shifts in key elements that have constituted the genetic body. Key elements of a post-genomic paradigm shift have been identified as entailing movement from: map-based gene discovery to sequence-based gene discovery; single-gene analysis to analysis of multiple genes and gene products in complex pathways or systems; structural genomics to functional genomics; experimental to biocomputational analysis; specific mutation-based genetic aetiology of disease to mechanisms of pathogenesis as complex process; collecting to implementing genetic information; and identification of genetic susceptibility to increasingly non-invasive monitoring of molecular changes indicating pathological processes (Peltonen 2001).

Of relevance for thinking about post-genomic bodies, this paradigm shift is envisioned to yield precisely targeted molecular intervention, expanding knowledge of interactions between 'susceptibility' genotypes, phenotypes and 'environment', movement of susceptibility monitoring further back in disease processes, and changing relationships among experiment and the human body. How will these shifts play out in conceptualisations of risk, responsibility, kinship, identity and governmentality?

The post-genomic body

The discussion presented here of possible contours of the post-genomic body is predicated upon scientists' visions of post-genomics as represented within key literatures and by key actors. Vision creation is integral to processes of technological innovation in the formulation of socio-technical networks and in shaping practices and artefacts, and has been prominent in the development of genetic technologies (Pinch and Bijker 1984; Martin 1999). According to Hedgecoe and Martin (2003), sociological exploration of technological expectations or visions, particularly for controversial technologies, should include attention to bioethicists and bioethical discourse as integral to the construction and shaping of technologies and socio-technical networks. Such attention might entail focus on:

Both the articulation of expectations in scientific and bioethical discourse in the form of specific visions, and their embodiment in the design of experiments and the formation of new biotechnology companies as a result of the decisions made by innovators. Visions therefore constitute a particular class of expectation which both project and anticipate how the future might emerge, and provide a strategic framework for actors as they attempt to construct particular socio-technical networks.

(Hedgecoe and Martin 2003: 331)

Scientists as well as bioethicists participate in the development and promotion of bioethical discourses and framings of technology; as discussed above, bioethics is increasingly enrolled by scientific actors and institutions as integral to the larger social processes of knowledge production.

The emerging vision of post-genomics is of multiple intersecting and heterogeneous socio-technical networks of knowledge acquisition supported by rapid technological innovation, occurring in parallel, hierarchical processes that are anticipated to converge upon systems-level knowledge about the human organism. The development of post-genomics involves the shifting of disciplinary boundaries and priorities – convergence of molecular biology, computational and materials engineering, chemistry, physics, and information technologies – and 'the development of new intellectual and physical spaces within which these events occur' (Glasner 2002). The latter include the establishment of institutes and collaborative projects dedicated to specific hierarchical levels and functions (e.g., Leroy Hood's Institute for Systems Biology, the Alliance for Cellular Signaling (AfCS), centres for molecular medicine established as interdisciplinary and biotech-spawning ventures at major universities across the globe) as well as integration across levels.

Like other heterogeneous networks, post-genomic technologies and knowledge production transgress putative boundaries among the natural, artificial and social (Wynne 1996). Emerging and envisioned examples of such transgression include: the introduction of synthetic DNA; nano-engineered and robotic devices as diagnostic and therapeutic modalities; the creation of new biosocial identities with prognostic and pharmacogenomic technologies identifying subcategories of 'treatable' or 'resistant' patients; the capture of human biological data/measurements – genomic, proteomic, cellular – in huge databases communicating through standardised languages or engineered 'ontologies'; or more grandly, the physiomic vision of a virtual human organism as mathematically defined, databased captured, within dispersed but linked model systems. The interplay, feedback, boundary transgression and reconstitution of nature, artifice and the social enveloped within these visions is staggering.

Convergence toward systems- and organism-level integrated science is being driven, in part, by imperatives to show benefits to public health from the 'big science' endeavour of the HGP, felt by both private industry and public funding agencies (Duyk 2003). The extraordinary promotion of genetic science has yielded a map, but to date relatively little in terms of therapeutic breakthrough has emerged directly from the HGP. While post-genomics promises significant breakthroughs in drug discovery, under current research and development processes the pharmaceutical industry faces both a high rate of failure in drug development programmes and a dwindling number of drugs leaving the pipeline. Finding solutions to these problems is framed by both government and industry as critical to public as well as corporate health, and is driving public–private collaboration in a massive research effort supporting multiple, parallel programmes to maximise the likelihood that viable products will emerge. Further, the much-touted promise of 'individualised medicine' may be unrealisable if such endeavours only diminish the size of potential drug markets without contributing to an associated improvement in the overall rate of successful drug development.

According to some within industry, and supported in the NHGRI roadmap, progress is hindered by 'the inherent lack of predictability of our available models for complex biological processes and the inability of our current life science paradigms to provide an effective road map for improvement' (Duyk 2003: 604). The major challenge to the life-science research community is to improve on its ability to reconcile molecular genetic research with integrative organ and organism-based research, to define 'clear chains of causality that would effectively "link genetics to physiology" in a manner that could form the basis for robust, reliable models of complex biological processes' (Duyk 2003: 604).

The promise of *predictability* based on system level convergence – on increasingly detailed and integrated knowledge of the human organism – is perhaps the most significant expression of the long-term vision of post-genomic bioscience. While currently distant, the vision has potentially profound implications for how issues of risk, the body, and ethics are reconceptualised. How predictability is defined, achieved and stabilised, and how it will constitute and be constituted within the post-genomic body, will be a key matter for ongoing situated analysis of post-genomics (e.g., Clarke and Fujimura 1992).[1] Stabilisation of systems-level predictability is being constructed as a 'do-able' problem, but will require achievement of coherence among material practice, instrumental models, phenomenological models and theory across multiple heterogeneous domains and actors (Pickering 1989, 1990).

Stabilisation, as is occurring through such mechanisms as the collective development of the Systems Biology Workbench, Systems Biology Mark-up Language, may serve as a far more potent platform for biological engineering than existing genomics. Some visionaries foresee in the stabilisation of predictability the possibility of changes in conceptualisations of risk, safety and evidence in clinical trials, resulting in mandated inclusion of simulation-based screening of therapeutics as part of drug approval processes.

Such an outcome would move the development of human therapeutics conceptually closer to engineering domains, where simulation and standardisation support requirements such as structural dynamics analysis (see, e.g., Kitano 2002).[2]

Post-genomic visions

I have selected two statements of vision drawn from different social worlds (clinical research and bioengineering) within the domain of post-genomic science that encompass different relationships among complexity, predictability and risk. While both posit human health, and more specifically drug development, as endpoints, the human organism, and thus the object of efforts to improve health, is constituted quite differently by each. For example, modalities (practices, materialities, risk concepts) through which the human organism is engaged as work object diverge sharply. In the clinical research vision, the post-genomic body is represented as the 'perfect experimental organism', enabled by molecular knowledge and the ongoing development of non-invasive monitoring technologies. More precise knowledge of molecular processes, with disease processes identified earlier and earlier in their development, suggest receding phenomenological risk to human subjects in biomedical innovation processes. In the engineering vision, the post-genomic body is both the source of model data and the object of model articulation and system simulation. 'Risk' emerges from data quality and standardisation, model articulation, computational complexity and distributed accountability – from choices and actions spread across sociotechnical networks. As post-genomic science progresses towards systems-level convergence, articulation among divergent conceptual, material and representational practices of the human body will likely be fertile sites for sociological analysis.

Both visions of the post-genomic body imply emergent forms of social relations and their normative regulation. Taken as potential alternative visions, they engage different notions of what post-genomic bodies, scientific practices and artefacts may look like, and the social relations that may emerge from and shape their production. And they engage notions of risk differently – the first, premised on a 'microethics' of risk reduction in human experimentation promised by molecular medicine; the second, premised on the expansion of risk awareness with the computational explosion implied by systems-level convergence. In one vision, risk remains a phenomenological property of bodies and subjectivities; in the second, risk is an emergent property of systems.

The perfect experimental organism

The first vision statement is from Dennis Ausiello, a Harvard medical professor and director of a pilot programme to train physicians in 'patient-associated science'. One expression of the paradigm shift of post-genomic science, as here represented, is a reconfiguration of the human body as experimental organism, knowable to an unprecedented degree in its complexity. The argument is predicated upon a vision of post-genomics, most closely articulated with functional genomics, as permitting precise characterisation of complex biological processes, an understanding that will both reduce levels of risk associated with human experimentation and increase the utility of addressing basic science questions within the environment of that complexity (the human body). This reconfiguration may be seen to be laying the groundwork or articulating with a reconfiguration of social relations among scientists, clinicians, patients and human experimental subjects with the goal of seamless translation from basic science to therapeutic modality. As with the genetic body, the body as human experimental organism is a metaphor for the social organisation of biomedical science, modalities of knowledge and technology production, and epistemic ends. Such metaphors may inform notions of experimental and therapeutic imperative, and govern the representation of risk.

> The mission to further the understanding of the human organism has addressed questions far removed from that organism. By necessity, the complexity and uncertainty that the human organism brings to any experimental environment have largely been avoided during the generation of new knowledge concerning biological processes. As we rapidly pass into the era of functional genomics, we are realizing the possibility of understanding and potentially intervening at the subtlest molecular sites of biological activity, as small as a single polymorphism in the human genome. Thus, we can now approach the human organism as a legitimate, even necessary, experimental model.
> (Ausiello 1999)

Echoing this vision of the post-genomic body, scientists interviewed in the clinician-researcher case study express great enthusiasm for the ability to link the actual patient body closely to laboratory molecular research within one investigator's stream of material and intellectual action. This enthusiasm is enhanced by the ability to bring together tools and materials in novel ways and towards resolving novel questions, but also to a belief in the receding risks associated with novel diagnostic or therapeutic technologies emerging from molecular techniques. The vision of the human body as perfect experimental organism, presented by Ausiello, is predicated upon the establishment of a partnership between clinician and patient around a work object that holds quite different meaning for each – the body. While raising long-standing questions of the ethical management of power relationships within clinical research (Sollitto *et al.* 2003), the notion that precise characterisation of molecular processes underlies more precise characterisation of risk facilitates the clinician/scientists interviewed to naturalise a commonality of interests and utilities with patients, even while they are of quite different character.

As research involving human subjects and more direct discovery of biological processes within living human organisms are perceived to present decreasing physical risk, the transformations of social relations within the clinic were not viewed by the clinician/scientists interviewed as presenting ethical concerns. The most potent changes in social relations in the clinic, as viewed by these researchers, were among clinicians and researchers themselves, in particular managing relationships across the traditional boundaries between clinical practitioners and bench researchers and conflicts of interest in the clinical testing of therapeutic modalities/ commodities.

All of the clinician/scientists interviewed, however, expressed a view of the ethics of their activities in terms of the existing paradigms of risk centred around genetic information. That is, the social relations and ethics of the genetic body in their visions map directly on to the emerging post-genomic body.[3] Ethical issues that were defined during the HGP era – information-based concerns of privacy and confidentiality, discrimination, genetic risk counselling, patenting – provide the framework for how the boundaries between science and society will be negotiated. Risk associated with genetic information is perceived to be undergoing refinement and expanding in clinical relevance to larger proportions of the population. As new types of molecular prognostic and predictive markers are identified for both common and rare diseases, issues of predictive risk anxiety, risk communication, and social risks including confidentiality and discrimination are seen as becoming more prominent features of clinical medicine (e.g., marker anxiety). The ability to identify patients with poor prognosis under existing treatment is seen as presenting both a new experience of medical futility, and a new manifestation of diagnosis lagging behind therapeutic development. Scientists engaged in clinical research activities tended to resist the notion of novel and emergent ethical discourses with post-genomics, and to stress continuity with but improvement upon current understanding of and ability to treat disease.

The virtual predictive organism

The second vision of the post-genomic body concerns the virtual assembly of 'scraps and fragments' of biological knowledge into integrated, dynamic systems. According to a website dedicated to the systems biology effort:

> The essence of system lies in dynamics and it cannot be described merely by enumerating components of the system. At the same time, it is misleading to believe that only system structure, such as network topologies, is important without paying sufficient attention to diversities and functionalities of components. Both structure of the system

and components plays indispensable role forming symbiotic state of the system as a whole. [sic]

(The Systems Biology Institute 2003)

The Physiome Project is a manifestation of the post-genomic vision of a complex, hierarchical, emergent systems-level understanding of the human organism in its environment. According to information provided on the project's website:

> The physiome is the quantitative and integrated description of the functional behavior of the physiological state of an individual or species. The physiome describes the physiological dynamics of the normal intact organism and is built upon information and structure (genome, proteome, and morphome). The term comes from 'physio'- (life) and '-ome' (as a whole). In its broadest terms, it should define relationships from genome to organism and from functional behavior to gene regulation. In context of the Physiome Project, it includes integrated models of components of organisms, such as particular organs or cell systems, biochemical, or endocrine systems.
>
> (Physiome n.d.)

The Physiome Project is an interdisciplinary, international, collaborative project for the interactive development and integration of models of increasingly complex hierarchical levels of biological functioning – a 'toolkit for the "reverse engineering" of biology' (Bassingthwaighte 2002). According to Bassingthwaighte, 'The Physiome Project is not likely to result in a virtual human being as a single computational entity. Instead, small models linked together will form large integrative systems for analyzing data. There is a growing appreciation of the importance, indeed the necessity, of modeling for analysis and for prediction in biological systems as much as in physical and chemical systems.' A number of biotechnology firms have already developed simulation products to model such processes as immune system response (e.g., Entelos is marketing a 'predictive biosimulation platform' called PhysioLab^{TM}). As with other efforts within the broader systems arena, these products approach future disease identification and treatment through model-based integration of many types of data to create emergent systems level understanding of human disease processes.

   In contrast to the vision of clinician researchers working on the molecular biology of specific disease processes, some proponents of the systems approach have appropriated an engineering ethic to a vision of the human organism as constructed through integrated knowledge products. Risk is understood as an emergent property of systems. Systems complexity, dynamics and emergence are associated with an expanded risk awareness of the consequences of intervening in an ecological model. Modelling, biosimulation and prediction bring with them awareness of the limits of knowability. The following statement, drawn from an article written by a bioengineer and proponent of the Physiome Project, places the systems-based post-genomic body in contexts of a macro ethical imperative to intervene, risk, and the technological search for predictability.

> Although we cannot predict the outcomes of drug therapy with certainty, we must go ahead. Despite the risk, designers of pharmaceuticals to alleviate AIDS or Alzheimer's disease, developers of stem cells modified to cure diabetes, and producers of materials for the prolonged, controlled release of drugs all have an obligation to move forward into the unknown. Every new bit of information reveals our ignorance of other information, and the maze of possibilities is impossible to fathom with the unaided mind. Computational tools for large-scale models are being developed and are anxiously awaited by biologists. Computers, even big, multi-CPU parallel machines, are still too slow to be much good as 'mind expanders'. We need computers that can answer our 'what ifs' in the time it takes us to think of the next question. Only then will we be able to critique efficiently the behavior of the models.
>
> We must do our utmost to predict well, not just the direct results of a proposed intervention, but also the secondary and long-term effects. Thus, databasing, the development, archiving, and dissemination of simple and complex systems models, and the evaluation (and rejection or improvement) of data and of models – are all part of the moral imperative. They are the tools necessary to thinking in depth about the problems that accompany, or are created by, interventions in human systems or ecosystems.
>
> (Bassingthwaighte 2002)

The author of this vision specifically links a 'macroethics' – an imperative to intervene – to govern systems biological efforts such as the Physiome Project to a macroethics motivating large-scale technological efforts for the 'long-term improvement of society', including engineering sustainable energy resources and avoidance of ecological disasters. The long-term improvement of society towards which the Physiome Project is directed is in healthcare – specifically, the imperative to pursue new technologies and new pharmaceuticals, the development of which involve placing some human beings at risk for the benefit of others. Guided by this imperative, and given the complexity of the human organism within environments of various scales, predictability of primary, secondary and long-term results becomes an ethical imperative. However, awareness of risk is heightened with increasing knowledge of complexity and the limits of the known. Predictability is limited by lack of information from lower, and up through successively higher, levels of biological functioning. The 'body' here, however, is not an organism but rather information, resident in interconnected databases and system models converging towards seamless integration and predictive capacity. The overarching systems task is overcoming, through processes of stabilisation and articulation, limits to predictability imposed not only by the current state of knowledge, but by the ability to engineer informational and organisational complexity.

The authority that a systems biological understanding of the human organism comes to hold within medical culture and its practices, human experimentation, and within the broader society, are matters currently for speculation. Like previous technoscientific metaphors and visions, it is represented as both tool and explanatory system, and presents properties (e.g., predictability) that suggest new and unprecedented forms of knowledge and control. The social power of genetic determinism was in the ability to 'read' what has been written in our genetic code – technologies have already been developed to make genotype information readable by non-experts. The flipside of predictability is its complexity. Individual genomes, even proteomes, are in post-genomic language merely a list of parts or types of parts with no indication of how they are put together. Functionality cannot be predicted from knowledge about each component. Assembling systems models and ultimately predicting functionality, and short- and long-term effects of interventions, is a collaborative, iterative and potentially powerful explanatory tool.

In interviews to date, clinician/researchers are resistant to the notion of relinquishing the phenomenological relationship to risk to predictive models, questioning the human ability to achieve sufficient understanding of biological complexity. They remain committed to phenomenological methods, and to advancing knowledge of disease and therapy, although with enhanced precision, efficacy and safety with technological innovations of molecular medicine.

A systems-biology vision of the post-genomic body built through human collaboration raises questions about limits of predictability (input, model choice) and politics (choices involved in modelling environmental complexity), including such questions as whose bodies and in what environments are the basis of normative models of system functioning, what gets modelled, what is asked and modelled about systems and environments, and how boundaries of the human organism are identified in relationship to what environments. Stabilisation and predictability imperatives also raise questions of accountability in collaborative database construction. Finally, the post-genomic body suggests issues of risk communication: how systems complexity will translate into clinical utilities that are communicable to human subjects, with what implications for trust. Stabilisation and predictability are also political processes, particularly as they become integrated into safety and regulatory practices in production of therapeutic commodities.

Conclusion

This new phase in the life sciences – post-genomics – is portrayed as necessary to bring the promises of the HGP to the benefit not only of human health, but of humanity in the broadest sense. Promises range from unprecedented understanding and control over the fundamental building blocks of all physical things, both animate and inanimate, to understanding and control over the broadest interlinkages and interdependencies of systems governing all life. Many observers have commented on transformations in the way science is now being done; however, there has been less attention to transformative visions of the body in its material, metaphorical and political senses.

The concept of the genetic body encapsulates impacts of the HGP on knowledge production, clinical practices, disease understandings, illness identity, concepts of risk, political choices and technology. It has captured emerging social relations, including relationships between bodies and governmentality. The concept of a post-genomic body may serve as a locus for similarly examining emerging transformations and impacts of post-genomics within science, medicine and society. Where genetic theories, methods and practices have been associated with reductionism and determinism (Kerr and Cunningham-Burley 2000), it is not clear whether the ways in which emerging emphases on complexity, interdependence, and constraints on knowability with post-genomics will reinforce these trends or move in other directions. Certainly the focus of individualised medicine appears to set the stage for increased precision, certitude and surveillance, and perhaps new technoscientific identities. The post-genomic body may be in transition from genetic inheritance and deterministic thinking to be increasingly constructed in terms of system dynamics, interdependence, instability and environmental embeddedness.

The systems nature of emerging post-genomic sciences, in which the interdependence and connectedness of life and environment at molecular, cellular, pathway, organism and environment levels forms the larger target of knowledge production and a central terrain upon which discovery science will continue, may require a correspondingly systemic approach to identifying and responding to ethics concerns. This analysis of technoscientific visions of post-genomics suggests that social processes of stabilisation of predictability in systems biology will be important areas to watch in the development of such science and the emergence of innovations. These developments may engender a convergence of biomedical and environmental ethics, both at a metalevel of action, risk and responsibility, and in specific instances of technological application. The traditional autonomy-centred approach to identifying harm and constructing ethical action in biomedicine may be ill-suited to systems sciences. Ethics is increasingly pushed towards grappling with complexity in the production of science and the technoscientific production of new individual and collective identities. This trend will only increase in the future.

Notes

1 For example, it is an open question the extent to which human organism–environment interactions and interdependencies will be captured in the

predictability vision of the pharmaceutical industry, or will implicate public institutions in the production of human and environmental health.

2 Ideas related to convergence and systems biology have a 'cultural life' as well in such works as Barabasi's *Linked: how everything is connected to everything else and what it means for business, science and everyday life* (Barabasi 2003). From this perspective, emergence would be a more appropriate term than convergence; however, emergence is too clearly part of scientific theories of complexity and thus, in my view, obfuscates the emphasis on the sociotechnical process of innovation.

3 For important analysis of how 'the social' has been conceptualised among genetic professionals, and the ways in which these professionals have constructed discursive boundaries between science and society, see Cunningham-Burley and Kerr (1999) and Kerr, Cunningham-Burley and Amos (1997).

References

Ausiello, D. A. (1999) 'Something for everyone: the human organism as an experimental model', *BBS Bulletin*, II (11). Available online at http://www.hms.harvard.edu/dma/bbs/bulletin/ june/index.html (accessed 12 July 2006).

—— (2000) 'Patient-oriented research: principles and new approaches to training', *American Journal of Medicine*, 109 (2): 136–40.

Barabasi, A. L. (2003) *Linked: how everything Is connected to everything else and what it means for business, science, and everyday life*. New York: Plume Books.

Bassingthwaighte, J. E. (2002) 'The physiome project: the macroethics of engineering toward health', *The Bridge*, 32 (3). Available online at http://www.nae.edu/nae/bridgecom.nsf/weblinks/MKEZ-5F8RKD?OpenDocument (accessed 12 July 2006).

Brown, N., Rappert, B and Webster, A. (2000) *Contested Futures: a sociology of prospective technoscience*. Aldershot: Ashgate Press.

Bruun, H. (2006) 'Genomics and epistemic transformation in the production of knowledge: the bioinformatics challenge', in P. Glasner, P. Atkinson and H. Greenslade (eds), *New Genetics, New Social Formations*. London and New York: Routledge.

Bunton, R. and Petersen, A. (2005) 'Genetics and governance: an introduction', in R. Bunton and A. Petersen (eds), *Genetic Governance: health, risk and ethics in the biotech era*. London and New York: Routledge.

Clarke, A. (1995) 'Modernity, postmodernity, and reproductive processes ca. 1890–1990, or, "Mommy, where do cyborgs come from anyway?"', in C. H. Gray, H. J. Figueroa-Sarriera and S. Mentor (eds), *The Cyborg Handbook*. New York: Routledge.

Clarke, A. and Fujimura, J. H. (1992) 'What tools? Which jobs? Why right?', in A. E. Clarke and J. H. Fujimura (eds), *The Right Tools for the Job. At Work in Twentieth Century Life Sciences*. Princeton, NJ: Princeton University Press.

Clarke, A., Mamo, L., Fishman, J. R., Shim, J. K. and Fosket, J. R. (2003) 'Biomedicalization: technoscientific transformations of health, illness, and US biomedicine', *American Sociological Review*, 68: 161–94.

Collins, F. S., Green, E. D., Guttmacher, A. E. and Guyer, M. S. (2003) 'A vision for the future of genomics research', *Nature*, 422: 835–7.

Cox, S. and McKellin, W. (1999) 'There's this thing in our family: predictive testing and the construction of risk for Huntington's disease', in P. Conrad and J. Gabe (eds), *Sociological Perspectives on the New Genetics*. Oxford: Blackwell Publishers.

Cunningham-Burley, S. and Kerr, A. (1999) 'Defining the "social": towards an understanding of scientific and medical discourses on the social aspects of the new genetics', *Sociology of Health and Illness*, 21 (5): 647–68.

Downey, G. L. and Dumit, J. (eds) (1997) *Cyborgs & Citadels: anthropological interventions in emerging science and technologies*. Santa Fe, NM: School of American Research Press.

Duyk, G. M. (2002) 'Sharper tools and simpler methods', *Nature Genetics Supplement*, 32 (December): 465–8.

—— (2003) 'Attrition and translation', *Science*, 203: 603–5.

Ellul, J. (1964) *The Technological Society*. New York: Random House.

Glasner, P. (2002) 'Beyond the genome: reconstituting the new genetics', *New Genetics and Society*, 213: 267–77.

Hallowell, N. (1999) 'Doing the right thing: genetic risk and responsibility,' in P. Conrad and J. Gabe (eds), *Sociological Perspectives on the New Genetics*. Oxford: Blackwell Publishers.

Haraway, D. J. (1997) *Modest Witness@Second Millennium. FemaleMan*™ *Meets OncoMouse*™: *feminism and technoscience*. London: Routledge.

Hedgecoe, A. and Martin, P. (2003) 'The drugs don't work: expectations and the shaping of pharmacogenetics', *Social Studies of Science*, 33 (3): 327–64.

Hunter, P. (2003) 'Putting humpty dumpty back together again', *The Scientist*, 17 (4): 20 (February 24).

Kelly, S. E. (2003) 'Public bioethics and publics: consensus, boundaries, and participation in biomedical science policy', *Science, Technology, & Human Values*, 28 (3): 339–64.

—— (2006) 'Towards an epistemological luddism of bioethics', *Science Studies*, 19(1): 69-82.

Kerr, A. and Cunningham-Burley, S. (2000) 'On ambivalence and risk: reflexive modernity and the new human genetics', *Sociology*, 43 (2): 283–304.

Kerr, A., Cunningham-Burley, S. and Amos, A. (1997) 'The new genetics: professional's discursive boundaries', *The Sociological Review*, 45 (2): 279–303.

Kitano, H. (2002) 'Systems biology: a brief overview', *Science*, 295 (5560): 1662–4.

Lippman, A. (1991) 'Prenatal genetic testing and screening: constructing needs and reinforcing inequalities', *American Journal of Law & Medicine*, XVII (1&2): 15–50.

Lock, M., Young, A. and Cambrosio, A. (2000) *Living and Working with the New Medical Technologies: intersections of inquiry*. Cambridge: Cambridge University Press.

Martin, P. (1999) 'Genes as drugs: the social shaping of gene therapy and the reconstruction of genetic disease,' *Sociology of Health and Illness*, 21(5): 517–38.

Nelkin, D. and Andrews, L. (1999) 'DNA identification and surveillance creep', in P. Conrad and J. Gabe (eds), *Sociological Perspectives on the New Genetics*. Oxford: Blackwell Publishers.

Parens, E. and Asch, A. (eds) (1999) *Prenatal Testing and Disability Rights*, Washington, DC: Georgetown University Press.

Parsons, E. and Atkinson, P. (1992) 'Lay constructions of genetic risk', *Sociology of Health and Illness*, 14 (4): 437–55.

Peltonen, L. (2001) 'The molecular dissection of human diseases after the human genome project', *The Pharmacogenomics Journal*, 1: 5–14.

Physiome (n.d.) Definition of the Physiome. Available online at http://www.physiome. org/About/index.htm#physiome (accessed 28 September 2005).

Pickering, A. (1989) 'Living in the material world: on realism and experimental practice', in D. Gooding, T. J. Pinch, and S. Shaffer (eds), *The Uses of Experiment: studies of experimentation in the natural sciences*. Cambridge: Cambridge University Press.

—— (1990) 'Knowledge, practice, and mere construction', *Social Studies of Science*, 20: 682–729.

Pinch, T. and Bijker, W. (1984) 'The social construction of facts and artifacts: or how the sociology of science and the sociology of technology might benefit each other,' *Social Studies of Science*, 14: 399–441.

Rabinow, P. (1992) 'Artificiality and enlightenment: from sociobiology to biosociality', in J. Crary and S. Kwinter (eds), *Incorporations*. New York: Zones.

Rheinberger, H. (2000) 'Beyond nature and culture: modes of reasoning in the age of molecular biology and medicine', in M. Lock, A. Young and A. Cambrosio (eds), *Living and Working with the New Medical Technologies: intersections of inquiry*. Cambridge: Cambridge University Press.

Rothman, H. (1994) 'Between science and industry: the Human Genome Project and instrumentalities', *The Genetic Engineer and Biotechnologist*, 14(2): 81–91.

Sollitto, S., Hoffman, S., Mehlman, M., Lederman, R. J., Younger, S. J. and Lederman, M. M. (2003) 'Intrinsic conflicts of interest in clinical research: a need for disclosure', *Kennedy Institute of Ethics Journal*, 13 (2): 83–91.

The Systems Biology Institute (2003) 'Systems Biology – English'. Available online at http://www.systems-biology.org/000 (accessed 28 September 2005).

Wynne, B. (1996) 'May the sheep safely graze?', in S. Lash, B. Szerszynski and B. Wynne (eds), *Risk, Environment and Modernity: towards a new ecology*. London: Sage.

5 Fashioning flesh

Inclusion, exclusivity and the potential of genomics

Fiona K. O'Neill

Introduction

Genomics offers us numerous subtle opportunities to fashion flesh. There is nothing new in wishing to repair, reshape or enhance parts of our bodies. 'Flesh', cutaneous, carnal, and now molecular and nano, was our first and continues to be our most intimate, yet social canvas. We fashion flesh not only so as to change our identity, but so as to belong. Flesh has become not only a material that can be fashioned, but one of fashion. Bodies are now dressed by and with modern technologies, as with clothes; where 'fashion sets the terms of *all* sartorial behaviour' (Wilson 1985: 3). Bespoke items have always been the height of fashion, whereas mass consumption has become the goal of fashion, even for flesh.

But what do fashion and genomics have in common? Fashion, as an act of manipulation and creativity, is what occurs with genetic material. But fashion, as a descriptive noun suggesting a trend that appeals and is usually transient, is not so obviously part of genomic progress. Yet 'fashion' as verb and noun are difficult to separate; together they form a conundrum and a paradox, as both exploit potential, often as novelty, in order *to fit and to appeal* – pragmatically and aesthetically, materially and socially. Fashion, in its exploitation of potential, is in effect part of the politics of progressive technologies. We may initially think fashioning flesh is all about cosmetic surgery, but if we look a little deeper we can find the influence of fashion throughout medicine. Genomics is offered up repeatedly as having the potential to revolutionise many medical practices; what must be considered is what fashionable influences will pervade such revolutions; what might we find hidden in the material and social potential we seek to exploit?

What might already be understood by 'fashioning flesh'?

Fashioning flesh automatically conjures images of cosmetic surgery; face-lifts, nose-jobs and implants. Guessing who has had what done to them has become an acceptable pastime, as has ridiculing those with surgical mishaps (celebrity plastic surgery websites), or watching TV series like the American show *Nip/Tuck*. Yet fashioning flesh is as ancient and global as the human race, though our motivations have changed considerably.

Since tools have been used, bodies have been modified: shaped, cut, reduced, augmented or enhanced. From binding heads and feet, to prehistoric trepanning of skulls, the medical folklore of Cosmos and Damien transplanting a leg (Barkin 1996), and breast implants, flesh has been fashioned. The body has been inscribed, from the Iceman of the Alps, whose tattoos some consider to be a record of acupuncture work, to the fashionably commonplace tattooing and piercing of the last decade. Prosthetically, false teeth have been used since at least the fourth century BC (Freeth 1999), false limbs now benefit from the use of computer technologies or a cadaver's limb can be transplanted (Jones 2002). The cybernetic hyperlinked electronic prosthetics used by Stelarc constitute performance art, as do the facial implants of Orlan.

The late twentieth century saw beauty move significantly, from a matter of aesthetic or economic luck, to one of idealised body designs sold as surgically accessible to the masses. Plastic surgery may have had its inception in World War Two with the reconstruction of battle-torn bodies and identities, but its coming of age began with the 'consumption' of cosmetic surgery in the 1950s (Finkelstein 1991; Bedell 2004).

As Shilling (2003) writes: 'In the affluent West, there is a tendency for the body to be seen as an entity which is in the process of becoming; a *project* which should be worked at and accomplished as part of an *individual's* self-identity' (Shilling 2003: 4). Whereas once bodies were ritually modified as a mark of belonging to the group, the body is now re-fitted or re-designed to be acceptable and/or challenging to significant parts of society and/or ourselves. Whereas body modification was once imbued with particular social, even sacred significance, as in a rite of passage, you can get Botox® at the hairdressers and a boob job in your lunch break. The now widespread preoccupation with youthful appearance and bodily performance perpetuates the emphasis on the body as 'becoming'. The aesthetics of appearance and the ergonomics of the body have been extended beyond asking 'what shall we do with the conditions for life that are given?' to asking 'what conditions do we want to order, today?' This is as a consequence of what is already on offer; as body projects move towards *body options* (Shilling 2003). Bodies as a given with 'natural' normative spatial and temporal parameters, like skin, allometric relational dimensions or ageing, have become mere flesh, an everyday manipulable material resource for all medical practices.

In his discussion of 'technoluxe' as 'a useful description of what neo-liberal medicine brings about', Frank (2004) outlines its dependence on 'the increasing public and professional acceptance of the body as something to shape and life as a project of shaping. It depends equally on the idea that projects are realized through acts of consumption' (Frank 2004:

21). Just as Featherstone highlights the influence of science-fiction cyborgs on business and scientific research practices (Featherstone 2000), similarly commercial cosmetic medicine can influence general medical practice and therapeutic research.

There is and always have been a plethora of reasons for fashioning flesh, some deemed necessary, others desirable. In the first instance, fashioning flesh can be an act of literally keeping the original body alive: where it is absolutely *clinically essential* to fashion the flesh, as for example in mastectomy to remove malignant breast tissue. At the other extreme the act is entirely *cosmetically elective*, where it is the individual who desires a change for no apparent medical reason: an augmentation of the given body, as with breast implants. Between these two extremes lies a third, significant, yet ambiguous area of the *clinically elective*. Here modifications are either made in order to treat non-life-threatening damage, to improve performance and/or appearance, as with breast reconstruction, or to enhance the performance and/or appearance of the original body on the grounds that there will be some broadly acceptable medical benefit, as with breast reduction to alleviate back pain. Of course the clinically elective may be utterly cosmetic and the benefits sought are psychosocial, as, for example, breast implants for transsexuals or breast reduction for obese men. These distinctions form a spectrum between what is considered absolutely medically necessary, what is considered medically desirable but personally optional, and what is considered medically possible yet may be said to be medically unnecessary, however desirable to the recipient. Across the spectrum there are numerous socio-ethical considerations, not least those associated with the formation or reformation of an individual's identity.

But why do we fashion flesh?

For many, the body is considered unfinished, vulnerable and leaky (Wilson 1985), and therefore it is in need of 'dressing'. Long before we viewed the body as 'a project of becoming', Socrates asked:

> whether our bodies are sufficient in themselves, or whether they need something else ... They certainly have needs. And, because of this, because our bodies are deficient rather than self-sufficient, the craft of medicine has now been discovered. The craft of medicine was developed to provide what is advantageous for a body.
>
> (Plato 1992: §341e)

There is therefore a certain sense of impropriety about the physical body, whereby it may need maintaining, finishing, enhancing etc., before it can be trusted personally and socially (Wilson 1985). Having faith in the propriety of one's body is fundamental to our self-esteem and therefore to our identity. This is where the physicality of *having a body* becomes part of *socially being a body*. As Crossley (2001) notes: 'The human body does not simply exist "in itself". It exists "for itself" too; as a focus of its own projects, concerns and contemplations. We inspect ourselves before the mirror, worry about ourselves; about our health and well being, appearance and demeanour. And we work upon ourselves to effect change' (Crossley 2001: 104). So, thanks to such efforts, we hope to belong in society within our social body, through our embodiment. Fashioning our flesh is therefore one way of expressing our personal sense of embodiment, our sense of how we belong in our 'self' and within society.

Hence, when it comes to an act of deliberate body modification – cutting the hair or the finger nails – it requires an objectification of the body as physical body, and can be viewed as a taking possession of the body, effectively as a social resource, such that in *taking control over the body* (Featherstone 2000: 2) we can become who we have envisaged ourselves to be: we come to belong to our 'self' within society – as our envisioned 'self' externalised. Yet we must not lose sight of what influences our sense of 'self'. Choosing how to belong, for oneself and one's offspring, is an ongoing negotiation of the tensions between one's sense of inclusion within a given or chosen group, and one's need for self-expression, one's sense of exclusivity.

We fashion flesh to overcome the vulnerability of the unfinished body in order to belong to our 'self' and society. We want, and maybe need, to belong to a group, yet wish like Winston Smith in George Orwell's *1984* to retain a degree of individuality (Orwell 1954). Considering why any individual or group fashions flesh engages numerous values in terms of our intentions, our prejudices, our self-perception and our understanding of how multiple others view us.

Recent events have put a focus on facial disfigurement as an issue which demonstrates the social engagement of medicine in deciding not only the boundaries between what is clinically essential and what is cosmetically acceptable, but also which body phenomena can be considered sufficiently significant to warrant novel medical interest and intervention. In doing this, our personal, social and material understanding of the body and its ergonomic and aesthetic ability/disability and normativity has been engaged and challenged.

Choosing how to belong: fashion and facial disfigurement

Let us initially consider a cosmetic example, elective aesthetic rhinoplasty: the 'correction' of the nose shape for non-therapeutic reasons. 'The first group of Americans to seek out cosmetic surgery in large numbers were Jews unhappy with their noses. Then through the 1950's they were joined by Italians, Greeks, Armenians, and Iranians, who were anxious not to look Jewish' (Bedell 2004: 1). Rhinoplasty remains a common procedure and, as Bedell says, 'Cosmetic surgery is a kind of political defeatism, a recognition that it's easier to change ourselves than to change the world' (Bedell 2004: 2). Significantly, this sentiment is echoed in Shakespeare's (2003) discussion of 'geneticisation' within the disability debate; quoting Parens: 'The easier it is to change our bodies to relieve our suffering, the less inclined we may be to try to change the complex social conditions that produce that suffering' (Parens, in Shakespeare 2003: 201).

But when rhinoplasty is used clinically as an aesthetic therapeutic, can it be disassociated from aesthetic social goals, as in the case of parents choosing rhinoplasty for young persons with Down's syndrome? This example demonstrates the blurring of the boundary between the clinically essential and the cosmetically acceptable (May and Turnbull 1992; Edwards 1997). The hope is for a better fit with, and therefore access to, society at large. There will be little or no performative physiological benefit from the procedure. The aim is to improve the Down's syndrome child's latent social potential and life trajectory. Here the motivation for surgery is one of normalisation towards a social prescription of suitable appearance, so that *the child* belongs; inclusion by being unobtrusive. Yet in this example one is led to wonder about the effect of social prestige and competition on parental decision-making. No one wants to see their child suffer in any way, including socio-economically. But, as the French saying goes – *on souffre pour être belle* (one must suffer to be beautiful) – so should the mentally disabled have to suffer physically to be normatively suitable? And for whom is this suitability sought? Is this act another transient socio-medical fashion, as with tonsillectomies and Caesareans? And are gene therapy or even amniocentesis immune: we see the number of Down's syndrome babies decline.

Second, consider the report in 2003 of the post-24 weeks abortion of a foetus with a potential cleft palate or lip. This case raised numerous issues; centrally the definition of what constitutes 'a serious handicap' (Day 2003; Dobson 2003 and responses). Has fashion played a role in this case? Childbirth is still undoubtedly socially prestigious and competitive. Understandably, parents want their baby to be as healthy, even as close to perfect, as possible. Parents face a choice between abortion, postpartum surgery, and non-intervention. Yet with the increasing availability and number of potential diagnoses through prenatal diagnosis, choosing to do nothing could be viewed poorly, almost as an act of deliberate disablement. The potential that prenatal diagnosis together with abortion offers a reproductively healthy couple could be viewed as a more socially suitable choice than that of postpartum surgery or living with their child as it is born. Is this indicative of a possible trend in the social-medical relationship, a transition from the creative manipulation of actual flesh through surgery, to the intangible fashioning of flesh through genetics, in time changing the face of humanity, literally and metaphorically?

Finally, a recent report by the Royal College of Surgeons (2003) confirms the feasibility of face transplantation using microsurgery, but highlights the considerable number of clinical 'unknowns' regarding final appearance and immunosuppression, suggesting a significant possibility for acute or chronic rejection that could lead to total or partial loss of the graft within the first five years. The report goes on to discuss the significant psycho-social difficulties that may be encountered by recipients and society alike. Yet it does not discount the future possibility for face transplantation, assuming the achievement of induced immunotolerence. This may be achieved through inter-patient gene therapy – the development of chimeric cells including stem cells (Starzl 2000) or through the cloning of recipient tissues.

Face transplantation has been considered because, for the severely dis-figured, the results of plastic surgery are considered by some to be insuffi-cient in restoring facial expression. Yet this has to be considered against consultant plastic surgeon Peter Butler's remark (quoted in 2003 in an online article no longer available) that 'The real crux is that this [face transplantation] is about quality of life, not quantity. You are trading a potential shortening of your lifespan against a potential improvement in quality'. The choice being offered is between quality of *potential* bodily appearance and performance, against quantity of lifespan, and con-comitantly knowing that if nothing else kills you, immunosuppression most probably will. You may be forgiven for thinking that this will never happen because cadaverous tissues is not transplanted for the sake of appearance, shortening people's lives as a consequence. But limb trans-plantation has happened, and it, too, is such a trade off (Jones 2002). UK and French teams have postponed their plans to submit proposals to research ethics committees following reports from the Royal College of Surgeons (2003) and the Comité Consultatif National d'Ethique (2004). (However, in February 2006 the French recipient of the first partial facial transplant attended her first press conference some two months following surgery; twelve potential recipients are being screened at the Cleveland Clinic in Ohio; and Peter Butler's UK team also has clearance to screen for potential recipients, though not to proceed as yet. It would seem that eighteen months is a long time in innovative medicine.)

Technically, face transplantation is about the potential of flesh, physio-logically and immunologically. The potential for psycho-social manipulation, offered by such organizations as 'Changing Faces' (http://www.changing faces.org.uk), has seemingly been put to one side to allow the technique to be developed. In this instance the drive towards innovation in plastic sur-gery through transplantation is the perceived inability to achieve facial expression, of not meeting normative aesthetic values for appearance and ergonomic values for performance. However, beyond this socio-clinical drive there are other factors to be considered, for face transplantation is involved in a 'race to be first' (Jones 2004). As a cutting edge technology it involves the participants in issues of competition and prestige.

It is important here to pause and remember that the overarching aim of the various Disability Rights Acts in the UK, Europe and the USA is to enable society to act inclusively towards those who are disabled. This is usually to be achieved by empowering the disabled with rights of access to the society of the able-bodied and its concomitant life qualities. In effect, this is an attempt to redefine the normative references of who can belong in society. Yet this act of inclusion, for the disabled person, should be as much about the inclusion of their expressed difference, as it is about access to sameness – whether socio-economic or surgical. This has been well expressed by Vicky Lucas (2003) and other disability activists and societies. The re-biologisation of disability, through genetics, now mediates this socio-legal move. Having moved away from disability as an issue of biological deficit for the 'limited' individual, towards one where the individual is considered 'impaired' by biological difference and 'disabled' by society's reaction to such impairment, we now see the possibility of genetics reintroducing the responsibility for impairment upon an individual, at the very least as their pathology (Shakespeare 2003).

In each of these examples, genetics may offer a potentially better solution to the physical problem, or a means to avoid it. Underpinning the choices on offer presently and into the future is the essential decision about how to belong with a given body: that is, how to belong to oneself and with others; whether to maintain an original sense of identity or to accept a new identity, materially in the flesh and socially in the reactions of ourselves and others. Hence, the medical options on offer will always address the on-going tension between our social need for inclusion and our individual need for a degree of exclusivity; with the current fashion for flesh and the body pervading both the individual's choice and the presentation of options.

The paradox and conundrum that is fashion. What is it really about?

'But it is always better to be a fool in fashion than a fool out of fashion – if we want to inflict such a harsh name on this kind of vanity; striving to be fashionable, however, really deserves to be called folly if it sacrifices true utility or even duty to this vanity. By its very concept fashion is a transitory mode of living.' So said Immanuel Kant (1974: 112). Kant is reflecting sentiments that still, in part, echo true. The folly of fashioned flesh is evident in the 'trout pouts' and 'wind tunnel faces' of cosmetic surgery's victims.

As Wilson (1985) notes, 'Writings on fashion, other than the purely descriptive, have found it hard to pin down the elusive double bluffs, the infinite regress in the mirror of the meanings of fashion' (Wilson 1985: 10). Fashion is paradoxical and a self-parody. The paradox lies in the emphasis upon novelty. Fashion entails change, through a rejection of the old in favour of the new, yet its own contention that *this new* is the ultimate resolution is soon undermined and contradicted by the *next* fashion. Fashion is also a fallacious expression of individuality, achieved through copying or directly referencing a rejection of others. The novelty of fashion is achieved only as a degree of exclusivity, to be shared with others, which is often short-lived. This ephemerality is what gives fashion it socio-economic status, its edge, in a world of mass production. We acknowledge that bespoke items have always been the height of fashion, whereas mass consumption has now become the goal of fashion, even for flesh. Yet fashion has been treated by the establishment as trivial, for established status *per se* is what fashion often mocks. The political power of fashion is embedded in its ongoing chameleon appeal to the consumer, and how it can mock the given status quo, creating that feeling of exclusivity to which corporate as well as private individuals can respond. However, rarely if ever can the investments made by consumers be fully realised, as time reduces such novelty to banality.

Anthropologically an individual (or corporation) may follow or refute a fashion depending on their need to display their prosperity and personal prestige, or as an indication of their personal freedom. Yet there are always normative references which one's expression of individuality addresses. These then define the groups to which one can or cannot belong. Fashion is deterministic. Yet it is the ability to manipulate these normative references, in a creative way, that allows for self-expression whilst accessing as many chosen groups as required. Beyond anthropology, fashion, and one's investment in it, reflects and engages the tensions between one's contradictory desires for inclusion and exclusivity. It also engages one's qualms about social suitability; the fascination and/or fear of, and the tendency for, perfectionism; which can lead to experiencing and expressing both xenophobia and depersonalisation – which returns us to Kant and the tension between the sacrifice of bodily utility in the face of wishing to belong.

When it comes to fashioned flesh, the novelty of research therapies is obvious. However, whether it is cosmetic or clinical, fashioned flesh is intended to be semi-permanent. Genetic therapies are for life. So how do these relate to transient fashion? Sweetman's essay about the contemporary body modifications of piercing and tattooing addresses this question of permanence and fashion (Sweetman 2000). Although some such modifications can be seen as little more than fashionable accessories, the relative permanence, and the investment of contemplation, pain and personal involvement, suggest that other modifications are much more than just fashionable accessories. Such permanent and semi-permanent modifications may even be said to constitute *anti-fashion*, which defines 'true fashion' as 'a system of continual and perpetual ... change' (Polhemus and Proctor, in Sweetman 2000: 52).

It is here that a clear distinction needs to be drawn between the permanence of an outcome upon the material resource being *fashioned* and the transience, or *fashion* trend: the styling. The transience of fashion is constituted in its process, not in its outcomes. A museum of costume demonstrates fashion not through individual items, but via the interrelated significance of the whole collection through time.

Clothing in and of itself does not constitute fashion, but novel transient styles of clothing do. So, too, a particular fashion may materially style the individual body permanently, but the process of styling, the trend itself, will not persist. High heels come and go, but the effect upon the body's pelvic girdle can be enduring, causing painful spinal curvature and difficulties in pregnancy. Medicine has its own trends. Tonsillectomies are out, hysterectomies and antibiotics are on the way out, caesarean sections, necessary and elective, are on the way in, the use of leeches is returning. There may be good medical reasons for these trends, none the less they are not disconnected from fashion. Each of these procedures permanently or semi-permanently modifies the individual body, yet, socially and within the culture of medicine, each goes in and out of vogue.

Socio-economically, for a fashion to be *the* fashion it requires an investment in novelty, and for each particular investment to be transient – for the consumer and producer alike. Such investments may in turn themselves become the fashion statement – as in the wearing of labels. (Anecdotally, a hairdresser told to me how a friend who, having had a 'boob job', focused attention repeatedly over several months on who her surgeon was and how much she had paid, rather than on the socio-physical results; similar anecdotes are told by those with hip replacements.) However, to further appreciate the multiple connotations of 'fashion' we need to consider the philosophical significance of the conundrum between the noun 'the fashion' and the verb 'to fashion'. In this sense, we are asking what is fashion-ing fundamentally about.

In essence 'fashion' is about continually harnessing *potential*. Potential is here constituted by two criteria reflected in fashion's role in defining what it is to *belong*, and in the *raw materials* with which fashion works, namely: *suitability* and the *manifestation of latency*. As a verb and as a descriptive noun the word fashion implies that there is a norm of performativity and/ or appearance to which one can and possibly should aspire. Significantly, all things that are manufactured are fashioned, they are crafted to be ergonomically and/or aesthetically suitable; *to fit and to appeal*. Consider developments in prosthetics, hearing aids, immunosuppressants; medicine aims to modify the body, and in so doing manufactures a 'new body' that is technically enhanced, potentially with non-original materials. Whether it is a 'good fit' or has 'real appeal', such fashioning is in the end about material and social *suitability*. Suitability suggests a norm, yet seeks an elusive perfection. This search for a quixotic norm is fundamental to the relationship between fashion's deterministic traits and its transience. Fashion is in effect the uncomfortable juxtaposition between the acceptance of everyday necessities and a preference for an illusory perfection of those necessities, ergonomic and aesthetic. As such, fashion is a driving force to progress in the making. What is sufficiently suitable today will be outmoded or banal tomorrow.

Yet we have come to associate the suitability of fashion merely with the linguistic modifier, as in *the fashion*, indicative of novelty, prestige and ephemeral values, engendering social competition and consumption – consumption which has invested significantly in the *fashionable appeal* of an item, potentially to the detriment of the *fashioned fit*. Here material suitability is in the service of social suitability, ergonomic fit becoming a poor second to aesthetic appeal. Yet it is the ergonomic fit, the material end product, with which one has to live, whilst the aesthetic appeal will fade. As Frank points out with reference to the cosmetic removal of small toes, 'What comes first is the shoe, which then dictates the shape of the foot. If the shoe does not fit, then perform surgery on the foot' (Frank 2004: 21).

Here we see the expression of potential in the manifestation of latency. Whereas potential suitability addresses how a fashion will engage with *what is*, the potential of manifesting latency addresses *what might be*. Fashion seeks out latency not only in the material fabrics with which it works, including flesh (as with the proposal for face transplantation), but also in social and personal values and desires. Manipulation of such latency leads to the manifestation of that which has not been explicit. It then appears as novel yet familiar, and so appeals. Originality in this sense is about a form of novelty, in which 'the new original' is sufficiently similar to its origins so that, first, it can be recognised, and second, it can be acknowledged as different but not *too* strange. When novelty is too original, too strange, often technologically, it requires other social or personal latencies to be manifested, to make it suitably fashionable.

This is how the dynamic tensions between suitability and latency motivate research and creativity. Such dynamic potential is what drives fashion, as a progressive influence on what could and should be, through the application of technology. Here fashion almost inevitably becomes pervasive, often insidiously so, as everything material and otherwise can be viewed as latent potential seeking to be made suitable. In its quest for more effective options, medicine is seeking out the dynamic potential in all other possible solutions.

So, the conundrum of fashion suggests that it requires an investment, not least of time and money, into novelty. When fashioning flesh, this is usually accompanied by a significant personal investment of physical and potentially emotional pain. Yet, however materially permanent the result of such an investment, it is unlikely to be socially or personally fully realised, due to the transience of trends. It is this socio-economic and potential material transience that generates further research and profits for the producer, whilst leading to the eventual economic and potentially social or personal detriment of the consumer. What makes genomics so 'fashionable' is its emphasis on the manifestation of latent potential.

Flesh, a surface with depth

An appreciation of 'fashion' having been outlined, it is only fair to give some time to considering what can be understood by flesh. All bodies, human or otherwise, can be seen as having a surface with depth. Each body is bounded by, and to an extent defined by, its external covering, its epidermis. Any depth beneath this defining surface skin may be a materially objective one, as in the depth of a damaged hip joint beneath skin, subcutaneous fatty tissues and musculature, when considering a hip replacement. Or it may be aesthesiologically, temporally, aesthetically and emotionally a more subjective depth, as in how various 'pains' are described when experiencing the development of an appendicitis. Just as with the body, flesh is not only an object of interest, but also a 'lived experience' of being, doing and being done to (Turner 2003; Leder 1999; Merleau-Ponty 1968).

Clinically, bodies are made up of fleshy parts: gross structural parts; limbs, organs, or finer material parts; differentiated cell types; cellular structures. Clinically, people need to be viewed objectively as an assemblage of removable, repairable or potentially replaceable parts. The relationship of one type of fleshy tissue to another from the same body (biochemically, histologically), or to the surface of that body (spatially, allometrically), or to another body (immunologically) can be assigned, based on certain scientific norms.

The lived experience of the body and its fleshiness is always a work in progress, of continuity, affirmations and uncertainties. The various depths of a lived experience come both from the social experience of the fleshy body and the personal experience of the flesh. As Leder (1999) demonstrates in his supplement to Merleau-Ponty's phenomenological conception, 'It is ultimately the body surface, visioning and visible, that is taken as the *exemplar sensible* of flesh. Yet this sensible/sentient surface cannot be equated with the body as a whole' (Leder 1999: 203). Leder goes on to make a case for 'flesh and blood' as a conception that engenders both the sensible/sentient surface, according to Merleau-Ponty's conception, and Leder's 'invisible' visceral experiences of the whole body:

> I know that the entirety of my perceptual world rests upon the unperceived coursing of my blood – if it were to cease, all else would cease as well. ... The liver experientially disappears precisely because it is *not* the origin of any sensory field. It does not disappear in the act of perceiving, as does the eye, but by virtue of its withdrawal from the perceptual circuit. ... Yet I am neither the observer nor the director of such occurrences. They unfold according to an anonymous logic, concealed from the egoic self.
>
> (Leder 1999: 207)

It is this 'flesh and blood' conception, juxtaposed with that of the material clinical resource, which needs to be borne in mind when considering flesh fashioning. For it is the phenomenological appreciation of flesh and blood that will experience the future banality of faded medical trends; whilst the clinical appreciation will understandably strive for more and better options.

Fashion, flesh and medicine

As demonstrated in each of the facial disfigurement examples discussed earlier in this chapter, there is an underlying tension between the *latent potentiality* of what could be done and what *suitably* should be done. Practitioners, by the nature of their work and under the Hippocratic Oath, are always seeking more latent and suitable potentialities. However, in doing this there is a real concern that medicine, its practitioners and recipients, becomes pervasively and insidiously embroiled in the socio-economic dynamics of fashion; in issues of prestige, competition, investment and their like. Often when we ought to be asking if *we should proceed* with this innovation, we find practitioners and others in fact asking *how we should proceed,* pre-empting any moral debate and thus fashioning choice from the outset (O'Neill 2003). Practitioners are understandably liable to fall foul of this conundrum through their enthusiasm and aspirations for their work. It has to be remembered that novel techniques offer not only the chance to solve once irresolvable situations, but to engage issues hitherto considered to be non-medical. In so doing they not only solve, but create, problems of medicalisation (Lesser 1988).

Fashion and genomics

If we take the defining terms for fashion we find they somewhat dauntingly echo the vocabulary of genomics: manipulation, creative expression, latent potential, suitability, inclusion, exclusivity, novel solutions, investment. This is not wholly coincidental. One of the foremost aims of medical genomics may be defined as creating *a bespoke technology for the masses,* as in pharmacogenetics. Remember that bespoke items have always been the height of fashion, and mass consumption has become the goal of fashion, even for flesh; so, what was once a matter of bodily luck holds the *potential* to become one wholly of bodily design. And if fashion and genomics are bedfellows, we must ask where we might find transience?

Medicine's quest for *suitable and latent potential*, and its concomitant continuing need for acceptance of such potential, is the same as that of any other social agent. Seeking more solutions that provide either the same solution more effectively or a different solution altogether is the nature of a progressive society. In this way genomics is an unexceptional inheritor of medicine's socio-economic practice of fashioning flesh. And, as with many present medical practices, genomics is subject to a Sorites paradox – function creep – whereby things progress from one practice to another such that incongruities, even fundamental changes, can go unnoticed due to the gradual continuity of such change. The philosophical referent is the ship of Theseus; the psychological referent the 'blindness' of scotoma. There is therefore an understandable seamlessness between genetic and non-genetic medicine, especially for practitioners. On a more practical note, latent potential is not a finite issue. There are numerous medical practices that cannot yet be given a definitive medical explanation of how they work, but they do work, and as such continue to be used and developed (e.g., Steensma 2003; Cohen and Leor 2004).

It is also important to remember that fashion is about a suitability which suggests a norm, yet seeks an illusory perfection; and that the dynamics of fashion are the tensions exhibited within and between *what is* and *what might be*. Historically the balance in medical practice has been firmly in the camp of living with what is; of 'what shall we do with the conditions for life that are given'; of returning the individual as closely as is possible to their original 'healthy' condition. However, the balance between *what is* and *what might be* is shifting. In part this is due to the move within the fashionable *body project* climate of cosmetic surgery towards a motivation for *body options*. This must be set against the public optimism that surrounds genomics (Palmer 2004) and related technologies. Both suggest a climate in which there is no longer an acceptance of the necessity of given boundaries for the fleshy body and the life which such boundaries determine. There is a growing sense in which the conditions we are prepared to live with can be ordered; potentially far beyond the life determined by the given fleshy body. Bearing in mind that, what is sufficiently suitable today will be outmoded or banal tomorrow.

In non-genomic medicine, the ends justifying the means thus far has provided relatively straightforward boundaries between what we could justify as being clinically essential, cosmetically elective and even clinically elective. However, genomic potential offers us something different. Although the vast majority of techniques that are presently being developed within genomics are for what would currently be deemed clinically essential procedures, the scope they will provide for elective medicine in the future will be considerable. Just as plastic surgery for the wounded of World War Two led to today's cosmetic surgery, what will tomorrow's genomics offer the fashionable? And who would have thought plastic surgery could benefit from a redefinition of death, as in the plans for face transplantation? The genomic aim of creating bespoke technologies for the masses may well challenge the present medical ethics means–ends justifications. When the necessity of the given boundaries for the fleshy body and the life which that determines are no longer central to our means–ends justifications in medical care, what criteria will then hold sway when multiple values are in play within a context that includes the thrust of fashion for transient novelty beyond the given?

Genomics is in many respects an unexceptional inheritor of the medical progress in fashioning flesh. What is exceptional, however, is the sheer breadth and depth of latent potential that genomics and related fields will offer within a nominal time frame, as a bespoke technology for mass consumption. It need not even come into fruition to change the expectations we have, the fashions we follow.

Conclusions

Although fashioning flesh would seem as old as humanity, the given boundaries of the fleshy body no longer hold sway over what essential or elective practices may be considered. The fleshy body has become a raw material resource, and in so doing it is reshaping its social connections and connotations. For it would seem 'technoluxe' is here to stay.

The body is a focus not only for our identity, but for our being and our belonging. As it comes to be viewed not only as flawed but as a work-in-progress, how we choose to engage with or escape from the suffering, prejudice and alienation some bodies encounter will be tested; self-perception and the views of others may well play a different role, in the light of what can or might be done to the flesh. Issues of inclusivity and exclusivity may well be further acted out on the fabric of the individual being, problematising belonging for us all. What genomics offers medicine, essential and elective, is a potential which matches the present enthusiasm of the body project experience and the fascination with body options. The fit and the appeal of genomics are thus captivating.

We are now at a point where we have to consider what will happen to means–ends justifications in medicine, especially those involving genomics; and if indeed the Hippocratic Oath is sufficient. Equally, consideration needs to be given to how the potential within genomics, not least as a social agent, may fashion our justifications for seeking the creative expression and manipulation of genetic potential. We need also to ask of medicine in general, what will decide the ethical criteria for inclusivity and exclusivity, for what will be clinically essential and cosmetically elective? And significantly, how are we to recognise the influence of transient fashions in deciding how we belong?

Acknowledgements

My thanks to Alan Holland of Lancaster University for discussing this chapter, and to Dee Reynolds of Manchester University for her communication regarding the expression, '*on souffre pour être belle*'; a commonplace French expression used towards young girls.

References

'Awful plastic surgery' (n.d.) A chronicle of celebrity plastic surgery. Available online at http://www.awfulplasticsurgery.com/archives/cat_bad_collagen_in_lips.html and http://dir.yahoo.com/Society_and_Culture/People/Celebrities/Plastic_Surgery (accessed 9 February 2006).

Barkin, L. (1996) 'Cosmas and damian: of medicine, miracles and the economies of the body', in S. Younger, R. Fox, and L. O'Connell (eds), *Organ Transplantation: meanings and realities*. Madison, WI: University of Wisconsin Press.

Bedell, G. (2004) 'How do you want me? Facelifts were once a Hollywood secret. Now they're advertised on the bus'. *The Observer Review*, 14 March.

'Changing Faces' (n.d.) The way you face disfigurement. Available online at http://www.changingfaces.org.uk (accessed 9 February 2006).

Cohen, S. and Leor, J. (2004) 'Rebuilding broken hearts: biologists and engineers working together in the fledgling field of tissue engineering are within reach of one of their greatest goals; constructing a living human heart patch', *Scientific American*, 291 (5): 22–9.

Comité Consultatif National d'Ethique [CCNE] (2004) 'Composite tissue allo-transplantation CTA of the face (full or partial transplant)'. Available online in English at http://www.ccne-ethique.fr/english/start.htm (accessed 9 February 2006).

Crossley, N. (2001) *The Social Body: habit, identity and desire*. London: Sage.

Day, E. (2003) 'Abortion campaigners welcome MP's change of heart', *Daily Telegraph*, 7 December 2003. Available online at http://www.telegraph.co.uk/news/main.jhtml?xml = /news/2003/12/07/nclef07.xml (accessed 9 February 2006).

Dobson, R. (2003) 'Review of abortion law demanded after abortion of cleft palate', *British Medical Journal*, (327): 1250.

Edwards, S. D. (1997) 'Plastic surgery and individuals with Down's Syndrome', in I. de Beaufort, M. Hilhorst and S. Holm (eds), *In The Eye of the Beholder: ethics and change of appearance*. Oslo: Scandinavian University Press.

Featherstone, M. (2000) *Body Modification*. London: Sage.

Finkelstein, J. (1991) *The Fashioned Self*. Cambridge: Polity Press.

Frank A. W. (2004) 'Emily's scars: surgical shaping, technoluxe, and bioethics', *Hastings Center Report* 34 (2): 18–29.

Freeth, C. (1999) 'Ancient history of trips to the dentist', *British Archaeology*, 43.

Jones, D. (2004) 'The haunting story of the incredible woman who could be given the world's first face transplant', *Daily Mail*, 19 June.

Jones, J. (2002) 'Concerns about human hand transplantation', *The Journal of Hand Surgery*, 27A(5): 771–87.

Kant, I. (1974) *Anthropology from a Pragmatic Point of View*, M. J. Gregor (trans.). The Hague: Nijhoff.

Leder, D. (1999) 'Flesh and blood: a proposed supplement to Merleau-Ponty', in Welton, D. (ed.), *The Body: classic and contemporary readings*. Oxford: Blackwell Publishers.

Lesser, H. (1988) 'Technology and medicine: means and ends', in D. Braine and H. Lesser (eds), *Ethics, Technology and Medicine*. Aldershot: Avebury.

Lucas, V. (2003) *What Are You Staring At?* BBC2, 6 August.

May, D. and Turnbull, N. (1992) 'Plastic surgeon's opinions of facial surgery for individuals with Down's syndrome', *Medical Retardation* 30 (1): 29–33.

Merleau-Ponty, M. (1968) *The Visible and the Invisible*, C. Lefort, (ed) A. Lingis (trans.). Evanstone, IL: Northwestern University Press.

O'Neill, F. K. (2003) 'Face transplantation: Is it *should we*, or *how should we*, proceed?', *Bioethics Today*. Available online at http://www.bioethics-today.org/FSarticles.htm (accessed 9 February 2006).

Orwell, G. (1954) *Nineteen Eighty-Four*. Harmondsworth: Penguin.

Palmer, S. (2004) 'The stem cell revolution', *Focus*, April (137), 24–30.

Parens, E. (1998) *Enhancing Human Traits*. New York: Hastings Center.

Plato (1992) *The Republic*, G. M. A. Grube (trans.), C. D. C. Reeve (ed. revised 2nd edn). Indianapolis, IN: Hackett.

Polhemus, T. and Proctor, L. (1978) *Fashion and Anti-Fashion*. London: Thames and Hudson.

Royal College of Surgeons (2003) 'Face transplantation: working party report', (chairman: Prof. Sir Peter Morris). Available online at http://www.rcseng.ac.uk/rcseng/content/publications/docs/facial_transplantation.html (accessed 9 February 2006).

Shakespeare, T. (2003) 'Rights, risks and responsibilities: new genetics and disabled people', in S. Williams, L. Birke and A. Bendelow (eds), *Debating Biology: sociological reflections on health, medicine, and society*. London: Routledge.

Shilling, C. (2003) *The Body and Social Theory* (2nd edn). London: Sage.

Starzl, T. (2000) 'The mystic of transplantation: biologic and psychiatric considerations', in P. Trzepacz and A. DiMartini (eds), *The Transplant Patient: biological, psychiatric and ethical issues in organ transplantation*. Cambridge: Cambridge University Press.

Steensma, D. P. (2003) 'ALG/ATG: illuminating the occult', *Blood Online*, 15 November, 102, (10) 3467–8. Available online at http://www.bloodjournal.org/cgi/content/full/102/10/3467 (accessed 9 February 2006).

Sweetman, P. (2000) 'Anchoring the (postmodern) self? Body modification, fashion and identity', in M. Featherstone (ed.), *Body Modification*. London: Sage.

Turner, B. (2003) 'Biology, vulnerability and politics', in S. Williams, L. Birke and A. Bendelow (eds), *Debating Biology: sociological reflections on health, medicine, and society*. London: Routledge.

Wilson, E. (1985) *Adorned with Dreams: fashion and modernity*. London: Virago.

6 Mapping origins
Race and relatedness in population genetics and genetic genealogy
Catherine Nash

Introduction

In March 2005 the National Geographic Society launched its new Geno-graphic Project – 'a five year effort to understand the human journey – where we came from and how we got to where we live today' (The Genographic Project n.d.). With the technological support and computa-tional expertise of its corporate partner IBM and the financial support of the Waitt Family Foundation, National Geographic's 'Explorer-in-Residence', geneticist Spencer Wells, coordinates this project to 'map humanity's genetic journey through the ages' (The Genographic Project n.d.). The online introduction to the project explains its focus on human origins, migration, difference and relatedness through the familiar trope of reading coded information about the past in the genes (Haraway 1997):

> The fossil record fixes human origins in Africa, but little is known about the great journey that took *Homo sapiens* to the far reaches of the Earth. How did we, each of us, end up where we are? Why do we appear in such a wide array of different colours and features? Such questions are even more amazing in the light of genetic evidence that we are all related – descended from a common African ancestor who lived only 60,000 years ago. Though eons have passed, the full story remains clearly written in our genes – if only we can read it. With your help we can.[1]
>
> (The Genographic Project n.d.)

The call for help here is to participate in the second of the Project's three strands. The first – *Field Research* – comprises the core of the project and involves 'the collection of blood samples from indigenous populations whose DNA contains key genetic markers that have remained relatively unaltered over hundreds of generations making them reliable indicators of ancient migratory patterns'. This will involve ten scientists in Australia, China, Russia, India, Lebanon, the USA, Brazil, South Africa, the UK and France, each covering a world region and carrying out local field and laboratory research. The second component, its *Public Participation and Awareness Campaign*, invites 'the general public' to participate in the project by paying $99.95 to have their own genetic material analysed and located on the project's developing map of human genetic diversity. Participants who learn of their own 'deep ancestral history' through the analysis can help the project by opting to allow the results to be added to the project's global database. The net proceeds of the sale of the Genographic Project Public Participation Kits will fund the third strand, the *Genographic Legacy Project* 'which will build on National Geographic's 117-year-long focus on world cultures' by supporting 'education and cultural preservation projects among participating indigenous groups'.

The Genographic Project thus represents one of the latest large-scale projects to map human genetic diversity. It also reflects the recent application of human population genetics in personalised genetic ancestry tracing (Tutton 2004). In the Genographic Project the genetic material submitted by 'non-indigenous' participants will be analysed by Family Tree DNA, one of the most popular commercial providers of genetic tests in genealogical research, at the University of Arizona. Companies selling genetics testing services for genealogy have capitalised on the popularity of genealogy in Western Europe and in countries of European settlement in the New World – Australia, Canada, New Zealand and the United States – and the scientific promise of genetics, by creating new genetic commodities for the genealogical market from the data and methods of population genetics. 'Personal interest genomics' is the term recently coined to describe the 'personal or recreational use of genetic ancestry information' (Shriver and Kittles 2004: 615). In the Genographic Project the methods of commercial genetic testing companies are incorporated back into a study of population genetics as a means of generating public interest and securing public support.

The Genographic Project thus represents the entwining of two areas of contemporary genomics that make direct claims to be able to tell us where we came from, and therefore in some sense who we are, as individuals, as human groups and as humanity as whole: population genetics and genetic genealogy. In this chapter I focus on the Genographic Project and Family Tree DNA to explore these two areas of science, commerce and culture. My questions are about the ways in which ideas of human difference, commonality, and connection are figured within these fields as they move between internet sites, newspaper reports, television documentaries, maps, material culture and science press. Genetic accounts of origin and relatedness have significant potential effects on the historical self-understandings and constitution of collective membership of groups whose 'myths' of origins are tested by population geneticists (Davis 2004; Nash 2006; TallBear forthcoming). The results of genetic ancestry testing may challenge, confirm or intersect with pre-existing familial, national, cultural, ethnic or racial identities (Brodwin 2002; Elliott and Brodwin 2002; Simpson 2000). As others have pointed out, recent developments in genetics suggest both the resurgence of racialised accounts of difference and new complex equations of culture, biology and genetics (Goodman 2001). Yet recent commentators, challenging earlier broad critiques of the resurgence of biological determinism and biological essentialism within and as a result of rhetoric of molecular genetics, have argued that people actively incorporate genetic information into their sense of selfhood and collective identities in complex and creative ways (Novas and Rose 2000; Rose 2001; Rose and Novas 2005; Wade 2002). New genetic knowledges, it is argued, are producing new active, informed and self-actualising forms of personhood and new communities and networks of obligation, identification and distributed expertise. But this creative incorporation of genetic knowledge and its dynamic deployments in the practice of identity and community coexists with the increasing reliance on genetics in legal cases concerning questions of collective membership, cultural ownership, rights to group benefits and, in forensic cases, identity itself. Furthermore, the effects of genetics on the dynamics of subjectivity and social relations are partly shaped by the sort of genetic knowledge in question.

Here I want to consider a particular form of genetic knowledge, its production and its lexicon of 'diversity', 'deep ancestry' and what I call 'genetic ignorance' in relation to ideas of geographical origins and relatedness: where we are from and who is related to whom? This involves considering its relation to the figuring of subjectivity, ethnicity and national belonging in popular genealogy. The growth of interest in genealogy has complex causes but in part reflects a version of subjectivity both forged and found through self-exploration – explorations of family history, as well as psyche and spirit. This model of the self, shaped through both the facts of genealogical knowledge and the process of uncovering those facts, intersects with the particular configuration of the categories of 'native', 'settler', 'national subject' and 'immigrant' in societies shaped by complex geographies of historical and contemporary migration. Both family histories of migration and reactions to new immigrants shape interests in ancestry (Nash 2002).

In this chapter I explore the ways in which the Genographic Project, with its avowedly anti-racist account of shared human origins, configures the meanings of human similarity and difference, connection and distinction. What sort of geographical imagination of human migration and mixing does it present? How is its 'public' constituted through its maps of genetic lineage and its participation strategy? How are people being invited to know themselves in new ways via genetic ancestry by Family Tree DNA and similar genetic ancestry services? In what ways is race refigured as well as avoided in attempts to construct forms of relatedness that make genetic kinship meaningful? In focusing first on the Genographic Project and its relationship to the wider field of population genetics, and second on genetic genealogy via Family Tree DNA, I trace the uncertainties and elisions that characterise the nature and interpretation of these technologies of origination as well as their more predictable effects.

Population genetics

The 'frequently asked questions' section of the Genographic Project web-site includes the question 'How does the Genographic Project differ from the Human Genome Diversity Project (HGDP) proposed over 14 years ago?' The answer given acknowledges the overlapping goals of both projects but stresses the differences between their aims and methodology. The website material emphasises the Genographic Project's basis in 'true collaboration between indigenous populations and scientists', voluntary participation and, through the Legacy project, plans to reward cooperation with fund-ing for 'educational activities and cultural preservation projects'. The website states that the genetic material will not be patented; the project is a non-profit-making venture; it is not linked to medical research and no pharmaceutical or insurance companies are involved. These assurances indi-cate an awareness of at least some of the criticisms of the ethics of the HGDP. In particular they avoid the charge that the extraction and patenting of bio-genetic material from indigenous groups is a form of bio-colonialism in which the value of their genetic material as a source of knowledge of human migratory history, potential usefulness to medical genetics and com-mercial value for the pharmaceutical industry is detached from any concern with the rights, welfare or livelihoods of those being sampled (Haraway 1997: 248–53).

Nevertheless, there are clear continuities both in terms of those involved – Luca Cavalli-Sforza, who proposed the HGDP, chairs the Genographic Project's Advisory Board – and in terms of the project's approach. Like the HGDP, the Genographic Project figures the genetics of indigenous groups as resources for understanding the history of human migration. Though one stated aim of the Project is to raise the profile of and empower indigenous groups, it is clear that their genetic material is seen as a threatened source of information. Reproducing the HGDP's fantasies and anxieties about purity and mixture, the Genographic Project figures globalisation and the 'mixing' or 'admixture' it entails as a menace to the task of mapping human prehistoric migration:

> Time is short. In a shrinking world, mixing populations are scrambling genetic signals. The key to this puzzle is acquiring genetic samples from the world's remaining indigenous peoples whose ethnic and genetic identities are isolated. But such distinct peoples, languages, and cul-tures are quickly vanishing into a 21st century global melting pot.
>
> (The Genographic Project n.d.)

Like the HGDP, the Genographic Project borrows from the language of biodiversity to stress the urgency of preserving human diversity (M'charek 2005). In this case the concern to preserve their genetics as a source of infor-mation about the human past is supplemented with a discourse of cultural preservation. Thus a multiculturalist celebration of diversity and a discourse of minority groups' rights to recognition and respect becomes distorted into an apparently progressive concern with cultural erasure. This concern comes with a culturalist notion of inherent difference that is at the same time biologised by genetics. It inherits also the HGDP's construction of genetically isolated, pure and homogeneous groups whose genes supposedly hold clues to particular events in the prehistoric geography of human migration (Lock 1997; Hayden 1998; Marks 2001). The stated focus of the project is on human migration and genetic interconnection, but nevertheless the construction of 'genetically and culturally isolated' indigenous people ignores the continuous history of 'mixing' that has shaped even those groups named as 'isolates of historic interest'. As anthropologists have pointed out, groups that may be relatively isolated now have not necessarily been isolated in the past (Lock 2001). The Genographic Project's focus on 'indigenous peoples whose ethnic and genetic identities are isolated' but are 'quickly vanishing into a 21st century global melting pot' unmistakably reproduces a primitivist fetishisation of purity. It contrasts a Western world of modernity and regrettable assimilation and a non-Western world of tradition and threatened isolation. The problematic paradox of 'the celebration of modern technoscience applied within the framework of archaic racialist language and thought, clearly loaded with astonishing archaic assumptions of primordial division and purity of certain large segments of the human species' that Jonathan Marks (2001: 370) identified in the HGDP can be found within the discourses of the Genographic Project too. But this project is also deeply shaped by a sense that the patterns of human demography shaped by prehistoric migration are being disturbed by globalised migration and mating. The hurry to capture genetic knowledge produces an image of the 'geographic promiscuity of modern life that resonates with the possibility of interracial unions and mixed-race offspring' (Wald 2000: 694). The Project is driven by a desire to map human prehistoric migration, but subsequent migration – after some unspecified point where everyone reached wherever they were going – is effectively seen as genetic miscegenation.

The theme of human migration is thus central to the project in both its fascination with ancient travel and its anxiety of about modern mobilities. But migration, especially when represented through the trope of the journey, is also used to authorise its accounts of human commonality and diversity. The Public Participation Kit comes with a DVD, as well as cheek swabs and glass vials, that includes the documentary 'The Journey of Man' produced by the PSB and National Geographic and screened in the US in 2004. It features the National Geographic's 'Explorer-in-Residence', Spencer Wells, and his journey in search of knowledge of 'our shared human journey'. The heroics of travel it features are both collective and individual. 'The Journey of Man' with its narrative of Wells's heroic adventure as 'lab-rat' turned anthropological field-worker following the 'ancient genetic journeys of humanity' presents a familiar image of Western, masculine exploration set against exotic people in exotic locations, one that follows National Geographic's long-established and visually luscious, primitivist celebration of diversity (Lutz and Collins 1993). Wells is on the trail of the genetic traces of earlier human hardship and heroic journeys in response to environmental change. Its storyline of prehistoric human groups struggling in their environments and setting out to new lands evokes an image of the pioneer founders of the New World, and resonates more specifically with the American mythology of the frontier. Yet the migrations being traced via genetics by Wells precede this modern migration and all that have followed by tens of thousands of years. In presenting the project as an 'effort to understand the human journey – where we came from and how we got to where we live today', the journeys in question are not those of European settlement, the displacements of slavery, nor the postcolonial migrations that threaten to cause genetic miscegenation, but prehistoric journeys out of Africa. This is far removed from the political economies of historic and contemporary migration. The public are invited to follow a shared human journey back to their origins, that may resonate with family histories of migration to the New World, but in ways that figure Africa as not only location of ancient origins but as place of the contemporary primitive. The 'public' that this documentary, and the Project more widely, addresses is unmistakably Western, defined against Africa as well as the indigenous groups that will be genetically surveyed in the Project. Evoking the image of a collective human journey and figuring Wells as heroic explorer, 'The Journey of Man' works to legitimate the Genographic Project's focus on the genetics of human difference.

But difference is ostensibly not the subject of the Project. Instead it is presented through the language of similarity. The newspaper *USA Today*'s report on the launch of the project, for example, included the statement from IBM's Ajay Royyuru, who heads the computer science team handling the project's data: 'The project is not about differences between people. It is about similarities shared by people everywhere' (Vergano 2005). The emphasis on 'similarity' serves to allay any concerns about the project's possible geneticisation, and by implication racialisation, of difference. Yet the central question and central hope of the Project reveals its concern with both difference and commonality: 'If we share a recent common ancestor, why do we look different from each other?' At the same time it hopes that 'the findings from the project will underscore how closely related we are to one another as part of an extended human family'. The Project's work on patterns of human genetic difference as a way of reconstructing patterns of migration that have led to human genetic diversity is repeatedly presented as a resource for global harmony and understanding. The Waitt Family Foundation, funding the Project's field and laboratory research, is involved because of its belief that understandings of difference can create harmony. Its website explains its ethos:

Where did the human race come from? How did we evolve to this point in our history? Why do we seem to look and behave differently from one another? Learning from our past is an essential part of The Waitt Institute for Historical Discovery's approach to making tomorrow's world a better place. We believe that if we can understand each other's apparent differences and their origins, it will become far easier to embrace what we all share in common and work together to promote a better future.

(Waitt Family Foundation n.d.)

This idea of understanding difference as a way of fostering a cooperative, peaceable world order supplements geneticists' claims to have done away with race. Population geneticists repeatedly argue that human genetic difference is a matter of gradients, and indeed many suggest that genetics has laudably disproved the idea of race as genetic distinction. Yet, as the comments on the destructive effects of 'assimilation' suggest, a desire persists for delimited difference, unclouded by the effects of modern genetic 'admixture' and the complexity of cultural categories. At the same time, this argument about the progressive effects of understanding difference does not necessarily come with much sensitivity to the ways in which difference is produced within the Project. The Public Participation Kit also includes a map that uses current knowledge within population genetics to plot the routes of human migration out of Africa and across the world between sixty and ten thousand years ago. On the reverse side the explanatory material is headed by a frieze of children arranged in a spectrum from light skinned to dark. 'Diversity' is ordered according the old schema of epidermal difference. The image uses the faces of children to invite the reader to enjoy this as an innocent image of innocent variety, but this is still a racial spectrum.

Nevertheless, the map is a map of prehistoric migration pathways not of racial variation. It is colour-coded to distinguish between the migration pathways based on paternal descent and on Y-chromosome inheritance from maternal and mtDNA inheritance. These blue and orange lines indicate 'the passage of a distinct genetic lineage' and are given specific letters and numbers. Yet, the principles of population genetics used in the Genographic Project are also being used by other population geneticists, and in other projects to map human genetic diversity that are more comfortable returning to a language of race. The Genographic Project is not the sole inheritor of the quest for the 'ultimate microphylogeny of the human species' (Marks 2001: 355). Numerous national and international projects are being undertaken which explore prehistoric patterns of human migration and the degree of genetic connection and difference between 'populations' or 'human groups'.

The crucial question here is what counts as a 'population' or 'human group'. Within population genetics there are two entwined approaches to this question: one which attempts to derive 'populations' or 'human groups' from patterns of genetic variation; another which explores the genetic character of culturally defined human groups, often in comparison with other culturally defined groups. The study of a Jewish Cohanim 'gene' (Azoulay 2003) and the work on the Jewish origins of the Lemba of South Africa (Parfitt 2003; Zoloth 2003) are the most well known cases, but they are multiplying as geneticists set out the solve 'myths' of ancestry and test assumptions of ancestral distinction. New maps of genetic diversity mask both the technological production of the 'populations' they delimit and the debates amongst population geneticists about the methods through which they are derived (Goldstein 2004). At one level this is about questions of sampling – of where and who to sample – and decisions about the statistical analysis of the data and where to draw boundaries within gradients of human difference. But the performative production of 'diversity' or 'human groups' involves complex and contingent relationships between objects, technologies, knowledges and agents. Amade M'charek's ethnography of the scientific practices 'consisting of individuals, technologies, language and theories' through which 'population' or 'genetic diversity' are 'enacted or performed rather than discovered, analyzed or animated' (M'charek 2005: 15) challenges the realist ontology of 'population' or 'human group'.

Some new maps of 'human diversity' suggest much more real categories of difference. The inclusion of the statement in the frequently asked questions of the Genographic Project's website that the Project has no connection to pharmaceutical companies, suggest concerns about patenting and profit that are the legacy of the critical reception of the HGDP. But it also points to the current research in population genetics and pharmacogenetics which focuses on the relationships between susceptibility to disease and patterns of human genetic variation. The aim is to explore the environmental and genetic determinants of disease and to develop drug dosages appropriate to genetically distinctively groups. The clinical usefulness of race and hope of advances in medicine is used to justify work by population geneticists fuelled by a desire to explore the correlations between ethnicity, race and genetic variation (Bamshad *et al.* 2004) and often funded by pharmaceutical companies developing 'ethnically' or 'racially' targeted drugs. The understanding of human genetic variation as relatively insignificant and graded rather than fundamental and absolute is orthodox in population genetics. Yet, population geneticists mapping human difference – sometimes inadvertently, sometimes assertively – reproduce racialised versions of human difference, some reverting to the old colour codes and classifications of racial taxonomy to draw boundaries within patterns of global genetic variation (Marks 2004; Sankar and Cho 2002). Though geneticists know they are convenient labels for what are effectively statistically derived boundaries within gradients of genetic variation that are themselves subject to the nature of the sampling and numbers of markers examined, these studies are then reported as genetically proving race. Even in less overtly racialised accounts the significance of genetic difference is inflated by the discourse of genetic essentialism and the promise of perso-nalised disease susceptibility predictions and prevention strategies, drugs and doses. This promise deflects attention away from the dominant causes of national and global disparities in patterns of advantage and disadvantage and the relationships between inequality, racism and patterns of illness, as it reifies race (Duster 2005).

The Genographic Project distances itself from the commerce of pharma-ceuticals and the language of racial difference. But the argument about the hopeful confirmation of human genetic closeness for the sake of global understanding masks the degree to which the Project is involved in produ-cing the difference it purports to be its subject. Difference is not exactly race here, but nor is it unracialised in the attempts to correlate genetics and culture. The 'anthropological genetic' work of the project will result in:

> The creation of a global database of human genetic variation and associated anthropological data (language, social customs, etc.). This database will serve as an invaluable scientific resource for the research community. Many indigenous populations around the world are facing strong challenges to their cultural identities. The Genographic Project will provide a 'snapshot' of human genetic variation before we lose the cultural context necessary to make sense of the genetic data.
>
> (The Genographic Project n.d.)

It is not clear how the 'anthropological data' will be used to interpret the genetic data. It may be that 'cultural context' means something about race. Those who buy the Public Participation Kit and who want to contribute to the project by allowing their results to be added to the global database will be asked to answer 'a dozen "phenotyping" questions that will help place your DNA in cultural context'. But it is clear that the Genographic Project sees its work as extending the application of population genetics into the study of culture as the term 'anthropological genetics' implies. Included in the Project website's news stories section is an account of an attempt to explore the effects of traditional tribal patterns of women's and men's migration for marriage on the degree of maternal and paternal genetic diversity within patrilocal or matrilocal societies (Maynell 2005). The implication is that knowing this genetic effect may make it possible to know cultural traditions in the past from the genetic composition of con-temporary populations. Population genetics can thus not only prove or disprove cultural 'myths' of origin but infer culture from genetics. The Genographic Project will track prehistoric population movement but, according to pages 18–19 of the Participation Kit leaflet, will also:

> Probe more profound questions: How has human culture – with its traditional gender roles, patterns of marriage, distinctions of caste – affected genetic diversity? Or, since linguistic and genetic diversity

mirror each other – both developing in relative isolation – what can our genes tell us about the origin and dispersal of languages? And, if we share such a recent common ancestry, why do we all look so different?

The Project's persistent focus on 'why we all look so different' is coupled with a lack of sensitivity to the risk that, by exploring culture's apparent genetic effects, culture and the social are geneticised and naturalised. The results of attempts to see whether distinctions of caste correspond to patterns of genetic difference, for example, could be interpreted as the genetic effects of social prohibitions of marriage between castes or read as proof of the natural order of structured distinction (Sabir 2003).

The Genographic Project has a way of presenting its work that makes it seem a world away from the sticky subject of politics. The children arranged in that frieze of epidermal difference are figures with the Project's family story. This is a trope that encompasses the intimacy of closest relatives and an imagination of the global human family. In the 'Journey of Man', Wells begins his travels by parting from his wife and children on a station platform. This family goodbye serves to emphasise both the solitary heroic and the sacrifice of his journey. But he also imaginatively brings his family with him as he explores genetic lineages of the human family and its migrations. Wells is filmed breaking the ice with San men by showing them the photo of his daughter in his wallet. The natural affinities of family are thus extended to a natural interest in 'deep ancestry'. Through the Participation Kit, the Genographic Project offers individual 'genetic lineages' and knowledge of the 'ancient genetic journeys and physical travels of your distant relatives', as it aims to complete 'the planet's genetic atlas' of human diversity. The explanatory material is careful to make clear that this is not conventional genealogy: 'Your results will not provide the names of your personal family tree or less where your great grandparents lived.' Yet the project is presented through the familiar trope of the human family tree. Participants who allow the results of their tests to be added to the global genetic database will 'help to delineate our common genetic tree, giving detailed shape to its many twigs and branches' (see also Wells 2002).

This is not conventional genealogy, but the project appeals through the genealogical pleasure of discovering who is related to whom, and the promise of surprising connections. Under the headline 'Tracing Humanity's Genetic Roots', a report on the project in *Business Week Online* included the following account of unexpected discoveries and possible connections:

Nick D'Onofrio has always been proud of his Italian heritage. The IBM senior vice-president of technology is a second-generation American, and his grandparents came from the boot south of Rome. So he was shocked when he learned in February that his ancestry stretched back to the Middle East's Fertile Crescent. 'Nobody was more flabbergasted than me at the news', says D'Onofrio. 'I said, "What? I'm Italian!" ... Now everybody else has the chance to trace their roots – and perhaps get a surprise like D'Onofrio. ... All sorts of connections can come out of this. Royyuru [head of the IBM research team involved in the project] can trace his roots back six generations in India. 'Beyond that, it's total darkness. I have no idea where I came from', he says. Before D'Onofrio knew his grandparents worked in Italy as a shoe maker and a truck driver. Now, he's aware of the Middle Eastern connection. He also knows that people with his genetic pattern swung through India at one point in prehistory. This raises the intriguing possibility that D'Onofrio and Royyuru are distant cousins. If you go back far enough, we're all related. Bringing that fact home in a fractious world may be the most valuable lesson that the project can teach.

(Hamm 2005)

D'Onofrio's response to the genetic analysis of his Y-chromosome type on his sense of identity as an American man proud of his Italian heritage suggests the ways in which the Genographic Project, like commercial genetic ancestry testing companies, produce personalised knowledge of genetic ancestry that inevitably intersects with existing senses of ethnicity and cultural origins, often in surprising ways. D'Onofrio is made newly aware of a Middle Eastern connection. D'Onofrio and Royyuru could be distant cousins. In this account the temporalities of population genetics are radically telescoped. Recent generations – two, three or even six – are far from the tens of thousands of years that distinguish 'genetic lineages'. If D'Onofrio and Royyuru are 'distant cousins', then this category of 'cousins' includes millions of other people too. These dissonant temporalities and this extended version of cousin kinship could make the claims of genetic relatedness meaningless. Do they then at the same time undermine the apparently constructive message that 'we're all related'? Inadvertently, despite the claims of its 'valuable lesson', these stories of making connections and revealing personalised deep ancestry reveal the project to be more about specific connections – and patterns of difference and similarity – than generalised human genetic ancestral interconnection. While these genetic lineages are geographically described rather than racially labelled in the Genographic Project, the results of the tests do not say 'we're all related' but locate individuals within a map of human genetic difference. The implication is that newly recognised global biological closeness will dissolve antipathy to difference. But the 'human family' is not an unambiguously helpful substitute for race. Since the family is a model of relatedness reckoned in terms of near or close connection, foregrounding biology as the basis of global harmony suggests diminishing empathy with increasing biological difference. The idea of the human family has been historically effective in producing and legitimating the hierarchies of racial difference that the Project wants to relegate to a less enlightened past. The trope of the family carries them forward.

In the Genographic Project, as in other genetic population studies largely concerned with prehistoric, or at least premodern population patterns, modern migration needs to be dealt with methodologically by focusing on 'isolated populations', screening out the effect of migration through sampling strategies, or developing techniques for calculating 'admixture'. Yet modern migration patterns, especially European settlement in the New World, create the cultural conditions in which genetic answers to questions of origins are so appealing. The Genographic Project taps into existing genealogical interests but it also constructs a new form of ignorance or lack that it then offers to rectify. The account of the commuter scientist who knows his genealogy in India back six generations but says 'I have no idea where I came from' produces a model of unknown genetic knowledge that had no prior existence as a lack. Genetic ignorance is thus newly manufactured as an absence of knowledge that needs to be addressed. Genetic ancestry tracing thus capitalises on and encourages what Donna Haraway (1997: 255) has called 'Epistemophilia, the lusty search for knowledge of origins'. How it does so, through reproducing familiar and generating novel versions of identity and relatedness, is the subject of the next section.

Genetic genealogy

Family Tree DNA, the company processing the genetic material of those who buy the Genographic Project Public Participation Kits, was one of the first commercial providers of genetic tests for use in genealogy. This is a new and fast growing area. Family Tree DNA was established in 2000 and there are now over ten US- or UK-based companies constructing and serving consumer demand for these tests. The launch of the Genographic Project in March 2005 coincided with two indicative developments – the publication of the first issue of the on-line *Journal of Genetic Genealogy* and the foundation of the International Society of Genetic Genealogy – one with the objective of establishing the academic credibility and professional status of the new field, and the other reflecting the efforts of consumers to develop mutual support networks as they use new genetic technologies and knowledges. Over the past five years this application of human population genetics for popular genealogy has involved the construction of these tests as desirable commodities and the manufacture of a culture of what is commonly described as 'genetic genealogy', but also as 'anthrogenealogy' (by Family Tree DNA) or 'genetealogy' (by one on-line information site and published guide) (Smolenyak Smolenyak and Turner 2004). This has involved situating these genetic services within the existing culture of genealogy. The Salt Lake City-based company Relative Genetics, for example, encourages potential customers to incorporate genetics into the legacy of genealogical knowledge that will be passed on to future generations. But, according to the Relative Genetics website, it also likens the tests to other new locational devices: 'In fact, you could say that DNA is a new kind of GPS – a Genealogical Positioning System'. Relative Genetics encourages the use of genetic tests in tandem with documentary genealogy, but this allusion suggests that with new technologies you can not only know where exactly you are and have recently been, but somehow know exactly where you come from.

More generally, the strategies of making these tests meaningful draw on existing categories of identity and relatedness – race and ethnicity, as well as the family. But they also involve attempts to construct new ways of knowing the self, new concepts of genetic lineage and new forms of genetic kinship. This double strategy of evoking familiar categories of identity and understandings of relatedness and constructing new forms reflects both the ease and the difficulties of incorporating the particular nature of genetic information into the cultures of genealogy. In marketing these tests, it is relatively easy to draw on the cultural significance of roots, ancestry and biogenetic inheritance, even if to do so requires stretching their significance to the extended temporalities of population genetics. But it is harder to invest the numbers and letters that name genetic markers and haplogroups with the resonances of genealogy's evocative names of dead or distant relatives. So how do cheek cells get technologically and culturally processed to produce meaning?

The samples sent to Family Tree DNA, care of the Genographic Project, by those who have bought the kit and done their cheek swabs, are analysed through two types of tests that are widely used in geneticised genealogy – Y-DNA (or Y-chromosome) and mitochrondrial DNA (or mtDNA) tests. The particular nature of the inheritance of Y chromosomes from fathers to sons and MtDNA from mothers to children have provided proxies for geneticists exploring patterns of human genetic relatedness. As the website genetic tutorials explain, in human reproduction the genetic contribution of each parent is shuffled to generate the genetic distinctiveness of each offspring. This is with the exception of the non-recombining part of the Y chromosome which is inherited directly from father to son, and mtDNA which is contributed via the mother's ova and passed on directly to children. This means that the mutations that occur over time in the form of Y chromosomes and mtDNA are also passed on, so that different direct paternal lineages and different direct maternal lineages can be distinguished from each other. Genetic tests compare key markers on regions of the Y chromosome and mtDNA that are known to be highly variable. Those sharing markers are judged to share direct material or paternal decent. The greater the number of markers examined, the more accurate are the results and more expensive is the genetic test. Though men can be offered information on both their direct maternal and paternal lineages, presumably to ensure equity, save confusion, and simplify the pricing structure, in the Genographic Project, male participants' genetic material is only tested 'to identify, your deep ancestral geographic origins on your direct paternal line'. For women, the mtDNA test is used 'to identify the ancestral migratory origins of your direct maternal line'.

However, the results of these tests are virtually meaningless on their own. Taking the form of a set of numbers for each of the markers and /or sometimes a haplotype letter, they are radically dissimilar to the conventional data of genealogy. Even if entirely decontextualised, the names and dates of birth and death of dead relatives give some sense of an individual life. These 'vital statistics' are usually enough to locate that life on a diagram of familial connection in the family tree. Genetic genealogy companies work to make up for the semantic emptiness of these numbers and letters by presenting them through personalised certificates, explanatory reports and sometimes maps. Their meaning can only be worked up comparatively – by comparing the results amongst people undertaking the test as a group, by comparing results with other users in commercial databases or by comparing the results with current global maps of the distribution of haplogroups and geographically coded databases of the results of population geneticists surveys, or ethnically labelled patterns of genetic variation.

Family Tree DNA explains that both its Y-chromosome and mtDNA tests 'allow you to identify your ethnic and geographic origins'. Consumers of both tests are offered the prospect of being informed of any possible identical or near identical genetic match to other customers whose results have been placed on the company database. If a match occurs and both individuals have agreed to have their details released, both 'Genetic Cousins™' will be informed of the match. No naming of collective identity is involved here. Genetic Cousins are left to interpret the meaning of this connection themselves, presumably by comparing the explanatory material they each have been provided with and trying to work out any possible genealogical connection. But customers are also able to view tables that list the country of origin of customers with genetic matches or near matches. These tables are the basis of Family Tree DNA's promise that genetics can provide information on 'ethnic and geographical origins'. 'Country of origin' here is self-defined. Those customers agreeing to supply information on paternal and maternal 'country of origin' are advised that, 'Unless you are a Native American or of Native American Ancestry, your Country of Origin is not the USA. It should be the country where your ancestors came from'. The combined genetic data and 'family origins' are recorded together on Family Tree DNA's 'Recent Ethnic Origins' database.

Nevertheless, the promise of knowledge of recent 'ethnic or geographical origins' is heavily qualified. According to Family Tree DNA, the problem is that testees may hold 'incorrect' knowledge of origins and that ethnicity is 'subjective':

> Incorrect origins provided by testees may lead to search results that
> do not seem logical. For example: Assume your ancestors are from

England, but your search results show the ethnic origin of your matches as England, France, AND one match shows an origin of Native American. Does that mean that your ancestors' relatives may have lived in England and France? Yes. Does it mean that your ancestor was also a Native American? No. This means that a settler in America had a child with a Native American woman, the child was brought up as a Native American, and that, over time, the family has 'forgotten' the European ancestor, and believe their ancestry to be Native American.

Over the span of generations people tend to move, as do borders, so nationality or ethnicticity [sic] becomes subjective. For example, testees may enter Germany for ethnic origin, because the land of their ancestors is Germany today, but the land could have been held by Denmark for many centuries ... Exact matches show people who are the closest to you genetically. The Ethnic origin shows where they have reported to have lived. Since many persons migrated over the past few centuries, you will typically see matches in more than one country.

So, despite strong offers of identifying 'ethnic and geographic origins', customers' self-defined Ethnic Origin, upon which this depends, turns out to be a very unreliable category, contingent on the vagaries of memory, migration, shifting borders, and the history of nation-states. But some answers are figured as more credible than others. In this explanation the surety and 'truth' of the knowledge of English ancestry is contrasted with the mistake of the Native American family forgetting the genetic legacy of a European male ancestor. Settler knowledge seems more reliable than the errors of Native memory. However, genetic genealogy involves much more active erasure. One crucial difference between conventional genealogy and genetic genealogy is that genetic tests only follow patterns of direct maternal and paternal descent. This double lineage for men and single lineage for women radically reduces what counts as genetically significant ancestry. Thus the dissonances between a customer's sense of ethnicity and those of other customers who are genetic matches can also be products of this reduction. A man brought up as African-American may be defined as genetically European because of a white paternal ancestor at any time in the near or distant past. Thus, though the account of the 'subjective' nature of identity in the explanation above seems to owe something to understandings of the historical construction of collective identities, there is a deeper essentialism at work in the reduction of ancestry to direct maternal and paternal descent and in the use of these patterns of ancestry to determine 'deep ancestral origins'.

In contrast to the apparent unreliability of self-defined 'ethnic and geographic origin', Family Tree DNA's genetic tests for 'deep ancestry' are presented as offering accurate locations within or outside named ethnic groups. The 'subjectivity' of ethnicity or ethnic origins here is replaced by the truth of genetically defined 'deep ancestry'. 'Deep ancestry' refers to apparently more reliable and genetically verifiable categories: Jewish, African and Native American. As the Family Tree DNA website explains, in addition to offering knowledge of genetic cousins, Y-chromosome tests for men will 'be able to check your Native-American or African Ancestry as well as for the Cohanim Ancestry'. The mtDNA test is 'able to indicate your Native-American Ancestry and which of the 5 major groups that settled in the Americans [sic] you are most likely to be descended from. It can also describe African Ancestry as well as other ethnic origins, known as the branches related to "Eve's Daughters".' But the reliability of these tests depends on a whole series of contingencies and approximations as well as on the assumptions that these cultural categories can be described genetically, and that the boundaries of membership are in essence biological. They are presented as not 'subjective' like self-identification, but they are deeply subject to the science of population genetics that promises certainty but performs its object of analysis from field sampling to statistical analysis to published results.

It is unsurprising but problematic that the companies do not reveal the degree to which the results are deeply dependent on the quality of their database (and the resolution, geographical coverage, sampling screening and delimiting of sample 'population' in the survey that produced it), nor the inexact nature of the science of the statistics of population genetics that produce approximations with varied confidence levels rather than the definitive answers suggested in the marketing of the tests. Despite lessons in molecular genetics, consumers are not invited to consider the process that produces claims to be able to test for a Jewish 'gene' – the starting assumptions, sampling strategies, statistical analysis and interpretations. In the case of the Cohanim gene a particular Y-chromosome marker found to be most frequent among men with the Cohen name is taken to be the marker for the Cohanim priestly group in ways which underplay the statistic shortcuts this entails and equate a cultural category with biological descent (Bolnick 2003, Marks 2001). Tests for African ancestry, like the Cohanim tests and all others based on direct maternal and paternal descent take less than 1 per cent of an individual's genome that the variable regions of the Y chromosome and mtDNA represent (Shriver and Kittles 2004: 612) as indicative of origins. The massive reduction of the family tree to lines of paternal and maternal descent is not made clear. The results are presented as linking people to the places and groups that their ancestors came from despite the ways in which 'migration within Africa over the past 400 years means that mtDNA and Y-chromosome lineages found in these populations now do not necessarily reflect those present at the time of enslavement' (Shriver and Kittles 2004: 612). The 'populations' or ethnic groups surveyed by population geneticists and assumed to relate to patterns of genetic variation are themselves more historically recent and more fluid than the offers of locating African origins suggest (Rotimi 2003).

Nevertheless, the possibility of recovery and restitution suggested by these tests for African origins is enormously potent. The deep political and cultural significance of African-American political projects of historical recovery in response to the historical dislocations and cultural erasures of slavery makes its difficult to challenge genetic tests for African ancestry. Critics who do, acknowledge that the appeal of these tests reflects the profound injustice of slavery and racism and the politics of historical identification and recovery, but argue against the equation of racial or ethnic identity with genetics (Baylis 2003). They point to the commercial motivations and divisive effects of genetically differentiating African-Americans into different tribal communities of descent, and raise concerns about the effects of geneticising ethnicity within African societies (Dula *et al.* 2003).

In their review of the nature, limitations and application of what they describe the 'estimations of personalized genetic histories', Mark Shriver and Rick Kittles argue that one solution to the reductive version of ancestry in Y-chromosome and mtDNA tests using 'lineage based analysis' is the alternative of 'biogeographical ancestry analysis'. Instead of tracing direct descent, this form of analysis uses:

[A]ncestry informative markers (AIMs, also known as population specific alleles (PSAs), ethnic difference markers (FDMs) and mapping by admixture linkage disequilibrium (MALD) markers) [which] are autosomal genetic markers that show substantial difference in allele frequency across population groups. These groups can range from relatively local clusters (for example Southern European/ Northern European) to larger continental distinctions (for example, African/non-African).

(Shriver and Kittles 2004: 613)

Family Tree DNA, like most other companies, uses 'lineage based analysis', but 'biogeographical ancestry analysis' is the basis of Print DNA's claim to be able to estimate a customer's ancestry in terms of the proportion of AIMs in the genome. The results are given as percentages of Western European, East Asian, Native American and West African ancestry. Here genetic genealogy is closest to that strand of population genetics seeking to identify and chart broad patterns of genetic difference between 'populations' ostensibly in the hope of developing ethnically or racially targeted pharmaceuticals. Shriver and Kittles acknowledge that the 'genetically defined ancestral categories that PGH [personalised genetic history] companies use could be misinterpreted as indicators of "real" racial divisions, even if they are explicitly acknowledged as being continuous and, to some extent arbitrary groups' (Shriver and Kittles 2004: 616). The source of this problem for them is the tendency to genetic determinism in the public at large and by some advocates and critics which the genetic testing companies need to combat. But as Deborah Bolnick (2003) has argued, their tests both misrepresent the nature of genetic variation and gene flow, reify difference and reinforce the traditional racial view of humanity divided into four discrete and isolated groups. The problem lies not in the public misinterpretation but in the very basis of the tests.

The persistence of such racialised imaginative geographies of human difference in one of the most popular pastimes in Europe and North America is disturbing. Even those companies who do not return to those four races via 'biogeographical ancestry analysis' align ethnic, racial and cultural categories with genetic descent in ways which play up the significance of blood and biology in models of human relatedness. Geneticists may discard ideas of discrete and genetically distinct human groups but retain deeply racialised versions of difference. It is telling that, in coining the term 'anthrogenealogy' to name the 'science of genealogy by genetics; especially: utilizing molecular biology to trace a lineage beyond the limits of historical records', Family Tree DNA defines anthropology as 'the science of human beings; especially: the study of human beings in relation to distribution, origin, classification, and relationship of races, physical character, environmental and social relations, and culture'. 'Anthrogenealogy' joins geneticised genealogy to a version of anthropology in which race is central.

Family Tree DNA thus offer two ways in which genetic genealogy can be made meaningful in relation to existing categories of ethnic identification, one using customers' own versions of 'ethnic and geographical origin' and one based on genetically-bounded versions of ethnic categories. In the presentation of these tests, the qualified reliability of the first contrasts with the confident reliability of the second. But genetic genealogy companies broaden their potential market by offering possibilities for developing new forms of genetic relatedness for those who are not interested in exploring possible Jewish, African or Native American roots. They do so by drawing on the existing cultural significance of patrilineal surnames and by attempting to stretch the meaning of maternal ancestry within and beyond recognition (Nash 2004). Since, like the Y-chromosome, family names in societies with patrilineal naming patterns are passed from father to sons and conferred on daughters and wives by fathers and husbands, geneticists have made much of the potential of Y-chromosome genetics to explore the degrees of relatedness amongst men bearing the same or similar names (Jobling 2001; Sykes and Irven 2000). Most popular genealogy is now not solely concerned with the male line, but the significance of surnames persists and is particularly shaped by their function in ethnically diverse societies as labels of ethnic ancestry and identification. Groups of people with interests in a particular surname and sometimes its variant forms, and often members of single surname societies, explore the genealogical connections between them, the name's geographical origin and the histories of migration that are revealed through the spread of the surname from this original place. Unsurprisingly, for many New World 'one-namers' this original place is in Europe. For some, the surnames are markers of clan

ancestry and surname studies are a prominent part of the popular genealogy of Irish and Scottish descent in the United States. At the time of writing (in August 2005), the website of Family Tree DNA states that so far it
has assisted in over 2,100 genetic surname projects involving over 11,000
unique surnames.

In the absence of a similar pre-existing cultural convention for tracing
maternal descent in the largely patrilineal societies of Europe and European
settlement, other sorts of work have to be done to make maternal genetic
descent meaningful. In the promotion of mtDNA tests this has involved
playing up a bond between mother and child and especially mother and
daughter, and deploying the biblical image of 'genetic Eve' and her
daughters. Family Tree DNA uses the language of Eve's daughters but does
not personalise the numbers which stand for mutation and haplogroups.
Oxford Ancestors, the main UK-based genetic genealogy company, has
gone much further by using its founders' mythologies of named and per-
sonified maternal genetic lineages (Sykes 2001). Customers are invited to
identify with those of the same maternal 'clan' – Xenia's, Velda's, Tara's for
example – via on-line clan discussion lists. These clan identities are ways of
generating senses of relatedness without recourse to categories of ethnicity
or race. Yet the value of genetic genealogy is often presented through
assumptions of the necessity for 'deep ancestral knowledge' and especially
the significance of its offer to locate personal origins in Africa for descen-
dants of slaves. This figuring of the value of the tests for those whose roots
are 'elsewhere' both draws on the significance of reconstructing Black
British and African-American history but can reproduce racialised versions
of national belonging (Nash 2004). The anti-racist reappropriation of the
mongrel and mixed as ways of thinking of national populations has to
contend with these new genetic differentiations of 'true' origins and genetic
distinctions between the national indigenous and non-indigenous. The
offer of origins elsewhere for some is paralleled by the image of genetic
continuity and largely pure descent for others. The Genographic Project
website's news stories section directs readers to claims based on genetic
and archaeological evidence that, '[d]espite invasions by Saxons, Romans,
Vikings, Normans, and others, the genetic makeup of today's white Britons
is much the same as it was 12,000 years ago' (Owen 2005).

While these attempts to generate meaningful genetic relatedness depend
on the existing significance of surnames, or extend the meaning of maternal connection to new 'clan' collectives, the use of new communication
technology in the making of cultures of genetic genealogy (both in marketing and consumption) suggest new forms of electronically assisted genetic
kinship. Using the technologies of databases and email communication,
many companies try to produce new models of relatedness that will give
meaning to test results that are not readily explained either by documented
genealogy, family memory or ethnic or racial categories. In addition to
on-line discussion forums organised on the basis of haplogroup hosted by

the commercial companies, databases are available for customers to search for and contact those who are genetically similar according to their Y chromosome or mtDNA. 'Y-base: genealogy by numbers' is a searchable database to which men can submit their Y-DNA results, their contact details and details of oldest known direct paternal ancestor, and search for near matches or 'genetic cousins'. Family Tree DNA offer similar public searchable databases – 'Ysearch' for men, and 'MitoSearch' for men and women – to which people can submit their results, search for matches and upload their genealogical records in the form of the standardised GEDCom computer files. These online databases that combine genealogy and genetics extend a recent culture of 'reuniting' from those based on former school friends (such as Friends Reunited) to genealogical connections (such as the UK-based on-line service 'Genes Reunited' for example) to 'genetic cousins' and 'deep ancestry'.

Commercial providers of genetic tests for 'deep ancestry' thus intentionally and inadvertently mix the seriousness of science and the playfulness of making connections. They combine the essentialism of genes and genetic descent as unquestionably meaningful with caution about the uncertain significance of the names, locations and numbers that appear as matches in genetic databases. The implications of the ways these tests appear to locate consumers in terms of deep ancestral geographical origins and in categories of collective identity depend on ways they are individually situated by the particular configurations of ethnicity, race and nation in different places. Genetic genealogy appears to offer certainty but its statistical estimates and approximations, and its stretched temporalities, are often incommensurable with familiar ideas of relatively recent genealogical connection and documented veracity. So the meaning of group relatedness via genetics swings in and out of sense and nonsense. It may be mobilised in politically significant senses of African or white European ancestry in the US, or be dismissed as meaningless. Genetic genealogy may offer pleasurable puzzlement or the wonder of genetic connections stretching across thousands of years and miles for some, but also have deep consequences for the senses of shared identity and group membership for others.

Conclusion

By linking 'personalized ancestral testing' and population genetics through its public participation strategy, the Genographic Project combines the two areas of genetics that make the strongest claims to be able to provide knowledge that has a direct bearing on personal and collective identity: ancestry and origins. This public participation strategy and its heavy reliance on ideas of the human family and human similarity reflect the ways in which racial science haunts mainstream post-eugenic human population genetics. This haunting is evident in the unknowing reproduction of primitivist models of the indigenous and the modern, in the fascination with difference, and in the readiness to biologise culture and human connection. But it is also apparent in the attempts to construct ideas of genetic self-knowledge and genetic relatedness that deflect the charge of racism. What emerges through this account of the new developments in population genetics and geneticised genealogy is not a simple return to race, though a critique of their most racialised versions is vital. Race remains the subject of some strands of research in human population genetics. However it is also both a problem and a resource in the work of others. Though some companies do claim to calculate racial ancestral proportions, much of the marketing of genetic genealogy is directed to producing forms of relatedness that avoid race but make the results of the tests meaningful, either by using a discourse of 'geographical and ethnic origins' or by fostering notions of genetic cousins through technologically assisted genetic kinship. Race is also a resource for promoting genetic genealogy. Many arguments for the value of population genetics and geneticised genealogy not only claim that they undermine race, but use the histories of violence, enslavement and cultural dislocation justified by racial ideologies to promote their potential to offer lost knowledge of origins and remake connections. The degree to which the public presentation of projects like the Genographic Project deploy an apparently progressive language of diversity, global human harmony, indigenous rights and cultural recovery in combination with a reductive version of identity, ancestry and descent is striking.

Though often constructed in ways which attempt to avoid race, ideas of genetic, biological connection and difference are threaded through the new forms of identity, self-knowledge and relatedness being constructed through the promotion of geneticised genealogy and population genetics. Companies like Family Tree DNA enlist the existing cultural significance of ancestry and origins in 'settler' contexts but they also work to produce a new need through figuring the absence of knowledge of genetic origins as a lack that has to be filled for the sake of self-knowledge and fulfilment. Genetic ignorance is a new condition, but it borrows from the cultural and political salience of dislocation and rootlessness. In constructing lack of knowledge of deep ancestry, the social recognition of the painfulness of the dislocation experienced by those displaced by war or poverty is extended to everyone. Everybody is somehow in exile, somehow originally from somewhere else. The narrative of human migration and survival that features in the Genographic Project resonates with histories of immigration and new-world nation-building, but does not necessarily lead to greater sympathy or understanding for the latest arrivals, or political engagement with the global inequalities that shape contemporary patterns of migration. According to the imaginative geography of human population genetics, modern and contemporary migration instead scrambles an imagined purity of people and place. Similarly, though the idea that 'everyone is related' is often used in arguments about the value of research in human population genetics, as this exploration of the Genographic Project and Family Tree

DNA has revealed, the research and business of population genetics turns out to be more concerned with making specific connections and differentiating lines of descent. The figure of the global human family foregrounds an apparently benign image of harmony, to frame the promotion of genetic tests for specific lineages as it obscures the real focus of human population genetics—difference. The speed with which the use of genetics in genealogy, and the idea of knowing the self and reckoning relatedness genetically are becoming normalised, suggests that this significant intersection between science and society needs urgent critical attention.

Notes

1 All further quoted material comes from the Project website unless otherwise stated.

References

Azoulay, K. G. (2003) 'Not an innocent pursuit: the politics of a "Jewish" genetic signature', *Developing World Bioethics*, 3: 119–26.

Bamshad, M., Wooding, S., Salisbury, B. A. and Claiborne Stephens, J. (2004) 'Deconstructing the relationships between genetics and race', *Nature Reviews Genetics*, 5: 598–609.

Baylis, F. (2003) 'Black as me: narrative identity', *Developing World Bioethics*, 3: 142–50.

Bolnick, D. A. (2003) '"Showing who they really are": commercial ventures in genetic genealogy'. Paper presented at the American Anthropological Association Annual Meeting, 22 November.

Brodwin, P. (2002) 'Genetics, identity, and the anthropology of essentialism', *Anthropological Quarterly*, 75: 323–30.

Davis, D. S. (2004) 'Genetic research and communal narratives', *Hastings Centre Report*, 34: 40–9.

Dula, A., Royal, C. and Gray Secundy, M. (2003) 'The ethical and social implications of exploring African American genealogies', *Developing World Bioethics*, 3: 133–41.

Duster, T. (2005) 'Race and reification in science', *Science*, 307: 1050–1.

Elliott, C. and Brodwin, P. (2002) 'Identity and genetic ancestry tracing', *British Medical Journal*, 325: 1469–71.

Goldstein, D. (2004) 'The genomics of race and ethnicity: the argument from population genetics'. Paper presented at the symposium *Race in the Age of Genomic Medicine*, BIOS, London School of Economics and Political Science, May.

Goodman, A. H. (2001) 'Biological diversity and cultural diversity: from race to radical bioculturalism', in I. Susser and T. Patterson (eds), *Cultural Diversity in the United States: a critical reader*. Oxford: Blackwell.

Hamm, S. (2005) 'Tracing humanity's genetic roots', *Business Week Online*, 13 April. Available online at: http://www.businessweek.com/bwdaily/dnflash/apr2005/nf20050413_6564_db016.htm (accessed 19 July 2006).

Haraway, D. J. (1997) *Modest Witness@Second Millennium. FemaleMan*™ *Meets OncoMouse*™: *feminism and technoscience*. London: Routledge.

Hayden, C. (1998) 'A biodiversity sampler for the millennium', in S. Franklin and H. Ragoné (eds), *Reproducing Reproduction: kinship, power, and technological innovation*. Philadelphia: University of Pennsylvania Press.

Jobling, M. A. (2001) 'In the name of the father: surnames and genetics', *Trends in Genetics*, 17: 353–7.

Lock, M. (1997) 'The human genome diversity project: a perspective from cultural anthropology', in B. M. Knoppers, C. M. Laberge and M. Hirtle (eds), *Human DNA: law and policy, international and comparative perspectives*. The Hague: Brill.

—— (2001) 'The alienation of body tissue and the biopolitics of immortalized cell lines', *Body and Society*, 7(2–3): 63–91.

Lutz, C. A. and Collins, J. L. (1993) *Reading National Geographic*. Chicago, IL: Chicago University Press.

Marks, J. (2001) '"We're going to tell these people who they really are": Science and Relatedness', in S. Franklin and S. McKinnon (eds), *Relative Values: reconfiguring kinship studies*. Durham, NC: Duke University Press.

—— (2002) *What It Means to Be 98% Chimpanzee: Apes, people and their genes*. Berkeley, Los Angeles, CA, and London: University of California Press.

—— (2004) 'The study of agglomerated human bodies'. Paper presented at the seminar *Biological Bodies*, Queen Mary, University of London, June.

Maynell, H. (2005) 'Women's travelling ways written in Thai tribe's genes', *National Geographic News*, 10 May. Available online at http://news.nationalgeographic.com/news/2005/05/0510_051005_genographicgenetics.htm (accessed 10 August 2005).

M'charek, A. (2005) *The Human Genome Diversity Project: an ethnography of scientific practice*. Cambridge: Cambridge University Press.

Nash, C. (2002) 'Genealogical identities', *Environment and Planning D: Society and Space*, 20: 27–52.

—— (2004) 'Genetic kinship', *Cultural Studies*, 18: 1–33.

—— (2006) 'Irish origins, celtic origins: population genetics, cultural politics', *Irish Studies Review*, 14: 11–37.

Novas, C. and Rose, N. (2000) 'Genetic risk and the birth of the somatic individual', *Economy and Society*, 29: 485–513.

Owen, J. (2005) 'British have changed little since ice age, gene study says', *National Geographic News*, 19 July. Available online at http://news.nationalgeographic.com/news/2005/07/0719_050719_britishgene.html (accessed 10 August 2005).

Parfitt, T. (2003) 'Constructing black Jews: genetic tests and the Lemba – the "Black Jews" of South Africa', *Developing World Bioethics*, 3: 112–18.

Rose, N. (2001) 'The politics of life itself', *Theory, Culture and Society*, 18: 1–30.

Rose, N. and Novas, C. (2005) 'Biological citizenship', in A. Ong and S. J. Collier (eds), *Global Assemblages: technology, politics, and ethics as anthropological problems*. Oxford: Blackwell.

Rotimi, C. N. (2003) 'Genetic ancestry tracing and the African identity: A double-edged sword?', *Developing World Bioethics*, 3: 151–8.

Sabir, S. (2003) 'Chimerical categories: caste, race, and genetics', *Developing World Bioethics*, 3: 170–7.

Sankar, P. and Cho, M. K. (2002) 'Towards a new vocabulary of human genetic variation', *Science*, 298: 1337–8.

Shriver, M. D. and Kittles, R. A. (2004) 'Genetic ancestry and the search for personalized genetic histories', *Nature Reviews Genetics*, 5: 611–18.

Simpson, B. (2000) 'Imagined genetic communities: ethnicity and essentialism in the twenty-first century', *Anthropology Today*, 16: 3–6.

Smolenyak Smolenyak, M. and Turner, A. (2004) *Trace your Roots with DNA*. New York: Rodale Books.

Sykes, B. (2001) *The Seven Daughters of Eve*. London, New York, Toronto, Sydney and Auckland: Bantam Press.

Sykes, B. and Irven, C. (2000) 'Surnames and the Y-chromosome', *American Journal of Human Genetics*, 66: 1417–19.

TallBear, K. (forthcoming) '"Native American DNA": race, and the search for origins in molecular anthropology', *Science, Technology and Human Values*.

Tutton, R. (2004) '"They want to know where they came from": population genetics, identity, and family genealogy', *New Genetics and Society*, 23: 105–20.

The Genographic Project (n.d.). Project website available online at https://www3.nationalgeographic.com/genographic/ (accessed 2 August 2005).

Vergano, D. (2005) '"Genographic Project" aims to tell us where we came from', *USA Today*, 12 April. Available online at http://www.usatoday.com/tech/science/2005-04-12-genographic-project_x.htm (accessed 19 July 2006).

Wade, P. (2002) *Race, Nature, Culture: an anthropological perspective*. London and Sterling, VA: Pluto Press.

Waitt Family Foundation (n.d.). Foundation website available online at http://www.waittfoundation.org/past/index.html (accessed 10 August 2005).

Wald, P. (2000) 'Future perfect: genes grammar and geography', *New Literary History*, 4: 681–708.

Wells, S. (2002) *The Journey of Man: a genetic odyssey*. Princeton, NJ: Princeton University Press.

Zoloth, L. (2003) 'Yearning for the long lost home: the Lemba and the Jewish narrative of genetic return', *Developing World Bioethics*, 3: 127–32.

7 The moral and sentimental work of the clinic

The case of genetic syndromes

Katie Featherstone, Maggie Gregory and Paul Atkinson

Introduction

Medical genetics services, like many clinical specialisms, are engaged simultaneously in the production of medical classifications or diagnoses, and the management of patient identities. Clinical work, such as is often glossed as 'decision-making', is therefore embedded in a broader repertoire of moral and sentimental work. The moral and sentimental order of the genetics clinic can be especially significant: the identification of an inherited, genetically-based medical condition has potential impact on social relationships of family and kinship; inherited medical problems can place in question the moral worth of parents; the diagnosis of a genetic condition can place in hazard the identity of a child. In the course of this chapter, therefore, we explore some features of this moral and sentimental work. The organisational context is a genetics clinic in the United Kingdom, and the particular focus is a variety of inherited syndromes that give rise to abnormal physical development and mental impairment. We explore how clinicians and parents co-construct the allocation of moral worth, individual and family identities in the context of clinical encounters.

There is now a substantial body of research examining the impact on clinical services of new genetic technologies, in particular the work of genetic counselling. The scope of this chapter does not permit a comprehensive review of this work (for overviews of the literature see: Evers-Kiebooms and van Den Berghe 1979; Biesecker 2001; Pilnick and Dingwall 2001; Wang *et al.* 2004). Areas of interest have understandably included the process outcomes of counselling: recall of information, patient satisfaction, predictive testing decisions and reproductive choices following counselling (Black 1980; Somer *et al.* 1988; Shiloh *et al.* 1990; Michie *et al.* 1994; Michie *et al.* 1996; Michie *et al.* 1997; Bernhardt *et al.* 2000; Collins *et al.* 2001; Barr and Millar 2003). Recently, there has been increased emphasis on the psychological dimensions of the clinical encounter (see, e.g., Kessler 1997; McConkie-Rosell and Sullivan 1999), the extent to which the principle of non-directive counselling is achieved (Elwyn *et al.* 2000) and the experience of counselling from the patient perspective (Hallowell and Murton 1998; Collins *et al.* 2001; Skirton 2001). Here, however, we are not concerned with the efficacy of counselling, nor with the interpersonal distribution of the genetic 'information' that is imparted on such occasions (see Featherstone *et al.* 2006 for a discussion of the latter topic).

More widely, the experience of parents who have a child with a disability or spoiled appearance has been a focus for research since the early 1970s (Brett 2002). Within that research tradition there exists an extensive literature examining the stigmatised identities of children with a disability. More precisely, parents' perceptions of stigma have been described for a range of conditions. Some focus on what Goffman (1968) terms 'discredited' individuals, in whom difference can be identified through their appearance. These include conditions such as craniofacial disorders (Hanus *et al.* 1981), Down's syndrome (van Riper *et al.* 1992; Prussing *et al.* 2005) and obesity in children (Latner and Stunkard 2003). Additionally, there are a number of studies examining families with 'discreditable' (Goffman 1968) members, where behavioural characteristics, although not immediately apparent, are potential threats to children's – and parents' – identities. These include disorders of developmental coordination (Segal *et* al. 2002) and epilepsy (Carlton-Ford *et al.* 1997). Studies have also examined parental coping mechanisms for 'courtesy stigma' (Goffman 1968), acquired as a result of a family relationship with a stigmatised individual, and one's identity potentially spoiled by association (see, e.g., Birenbaum 1992; Gray 2002; Norvilitis *et al.* 2002; Green 2003; McKeever and Miller 2004). We draw particularly on this body of work in this chapter, in the course of our discussion of parental perceptions of stigma and the sentimental work performed in the genetics clinic. These issues are of particular significance in the context of dysmorphology and medical genetics. We introduce the background to dysmorphology in the next section.

Dysmorphology

Dysmorphology is the professional discipline of delineating disorders affecting the physical development of the individual, before or after birth, and includes the recognition of physical features in patients with a variety of different problems (Aase 1990). The specialism has been described as 'the study of disordered development' (Harper 1998: 83). It includes the recognition of characteristic patterns of physical features and the identification of underlying systemic abnormalities. Some physical features may be associated with abnormalities but may not be entirely abnormal in themselves. For example, small ears may not be 'abnormal' in themselves, but may be part of a pattern of abnormal development in association with other physical signs. Such patterns of physical features are associated with underlying systemic abnormalities, such as heart defects or delayed intellectual development. When patterns of malformations are deemed to have reached a level of regularity across different cases and are thought to arise from a single underlying pathogenetic mechanism, they are named as a *syndrome*. There are several thousand named syndromes currently held within international clinical databases and textbooks (Jones 1997). Patients seen in clinics are mainly babies, children, teenagers and young adults, and clearly the parents of children and young people are thoroughly involved in the social processes of consultation, diagnosis and management in dysmorphology.

The majority of syndromes have been identified as having a genetic basis, which are either single gene defects or chromosomal disorders. Chromosomal abnormalities are spontaneous, *de novo* occurrences. When this is believed to be the cause of a child's condition, the risk of recurrence within the family is assessed as being low, particularly where no abnormality is present in a parent (Harper 1998). However, some syndromes are familial conditions as a consequence of an inherited genetic defect. If this is the case and the clinic can identify the underlying genetic constitution, then families can be provided with an estimate of the likely risk of recurrence in future pregnancies.

Dysmorphia in children clearly throws into relief the topic of identity-work within the clinical genetics setting. Dysmorphia gives rise to actual or potential threats to the attributed identity of the child, through the implications of spoiled appearance (Goffman 1968). In addition, because it is implicated in *genetic* medicine, this creates the potential for moral threats to the parents' identities and it is to this subject that we now turn. It is in the nature of genetic conditions that medical conditions and risks can have significant implications for other family members. A child with an inherited syndrome, therefore, may be felt to create identity problems for parents, siblings and other members of the kindred.

We draw on a one-year ethnography of interactional processes in the dysmorphology clinic. Observations of family–clinician interactions in specialist clinics and subsequent interviews with a sub-set of parents and – where appropriate and possible – patients have been carried out. We have thus been able to document a series of parental consultations in the clinic and the reported experiences of parents of their attendance. Some of these overlap, and where this occurs our analysis reflects the marriage of two sets of data: the observed, and the reported, experience.

The research

For the purposes of this ethnographic study, one clinical genetics team and their patient population were followed over a period of nine months. Thirty-seven consultations were observed in genetic medicine clinics based in three local hospitals. Although the caseload of the clinical team was not dedicated to dysmorphology cases, a large proportion of cases referred to them involved dysmorphology. The average length of time allocated to each clinic consultation was one hour. These are very different kinds of consultation from the fleeting encounters characteristic of most primary care settings, such as GP surgeries. The thirty-seven consultations studied equated to forty-four hours of observation. We also observed six local professional dysmorphology meetings where cases were presented and discussed by multidisciplinary specialist teams of professionals. In addition, a large number of less formal encounters between professionals was observed. In the course of the clinic study, sixteen patients and/or their parents agreed to be interviewed. The interviews allowed us to explore the personal and familial consequences of these diagnostic processes and our informants' experiences of the management of dysmorphia by the genetics service. In total, twenty-six people were interviewed. These referrals represent a range of stages in the diagnostic process.

The moral and sentimental work of the clinic

Some parents received a diagnosis of a named syndrome associated with their child's condition relatively quickly, once they had been referred to the clinical genetics service. However, for the majority, the process of attendance at the clinic and the search for a diagnosis continued over a number of years. In addition, referral did not always result in an unequivocal diagnosis of a named syndrome, and in such cases parents were usually provided with a number of potential syndromes that might be the cause of their child's disabilities, or were provided with the likely aetiology and the risk of recurrence.

The clinic provides a confessional space where parental concerns about the aetiology of their child's condition can be discussed and where the clinical team can attend to parental feelings of blame and responsibility for having 'caused' their child's condition in some way. The process of referral to the clinic involves the clinical team scrutinising not only the patient, but also the patient's parents and wider family members, for clues that may help to identify the cause of the child's disabilities (for further elaboration see Featherstone *et al.* 2005). For many parents, their referral to the genetics clinic, and its association with inherited 'familial' conditions, meant that they scrutinised other family members for an associated disorder. For example, a mother recounts her child's referral to a London specialist who asked whether they had been referred to the local genetics service. The mother recalls her alarm and anxiety at the suggestion that the condition might have a genetic basis. Discovering that 'genetics' could be involved provoked the fear that she or her husband, by combining their genes, had caused their child's problems:

> I mean if someone's got a genetics problem it's hereditary and it is something that Ross [husband] and I had done together and it was obviously very, very scary.
>
> (Son with Proteus Syndrome: *de novo* mutation)

Because a genetic diagnosis has the potential to identify the origins of the condition the clinic is a site in which blame and responsibility for transmission can be attributed. The genetic nature of the referral often led to parental (and wider familial) concerns that they must have contributed in some way, particularly through an act or omission during the pregnancy that had 'caused' or allowed this genetic change to occur. For example, at three points in her interview a mother discusses how she could have caused her son's condition; looking at the early stages of her pregnancy and also at her experience of labour as potential causes:

> What happened was a couple of weeks after I conceived him, where I went wrong, I racked my brains to see, but you know I didn't do anything wrong, I didn't hurt myself or anything so … I was thirty-six hours in labour and he didn't want to come out, but I mean they class it as a normal labour, I don't. But I wondered if something went wrong there. … I was like 'Oh God,' you know 'is this my fault?' you know? And for a while I was like, 'Did I have something, eat some bad food or, you know …'
>
> (Son with undiagnosed multiple developmental problems)

Parental surveillance also extended to the wider family (Featherstone *et al.* 2006). Parents reported examining their family history and other family members for similar problems that might indicate the familial origins of their child's condition. For some parents, the identification of a genetic cause for their child's condition enabled them to attach these feelings of blame to a specific family member, usually a parent, grandparent or a 'side' of the family. In the next example the consultant provides parents with a diagnosis of polymicrogyria (associated with developmental delay, seizures and decreased muscle tone which delays development of infant motor milestones such as head support and sitting. Later this is evident from a slumped sitting posture, late walking and an abnormal gait. It is associated with a *de novo*, spontaneous mutation) for their son's condition, and reassures them that although it is a genetic condition it is not familial, and thus the chance of recurrence in future pregnancies is 'low'. However, this does not provide these parents with complete reassurance. They find it hard to believe the condition could have been a random event; and the mother focuses on her husband's 'side' of the family. She also describes how she continually questions whether she herself had caused her child's condition in some way:

MOTHER: Is it genetic?
CONSULTANT GENETICIST: Yes, but so far we don't think it runs in families.
    A gene is involved and early in the development
[…]
FATHER: It's funny, it's come from nowhere.

CONSULTANT GENETICIST: Which part of the family were you worried about?

MOTHER: His side, his mother and his sister's children, we've not asked them about it, it's difficult.

[They discuss the risk of this condition affecting future pregnancies and the diagnosis.]

SPECIALIST NURSE: Do you feel all your questions have been answered?

MOTHER: The 'why' question is always in my mind, having had the baby, did I do anything?

(Clinic 4, patient 1)

What is noticeable here is that the parents' spoken interpretations do not accommodate the purely random nature of the genetic event. They seek simultaneously for reasons in the family history and in personal behaviour in order to make sense of it. Issues of responsibility and possible culpability enter into their vocabularies of explanation.

The attribution of responsibility is not a one-way process. Not only can parents of an affected child look for causes in other family members, they can also be the object of familial scrutiny. Parents reported that other family members could also attribute responsibility to them. This came usually from the child's grandparents, who blamed their offspring's partner for causing or passing on the condition in some way. Most commonly, mothers recounted stories – both within the clinical setting and during interviews at home – of being identified as the likely source of their child's problems, by passing on a familial problem or through acts or omissions during the pregnancy itself.

While genetic conditions give rise to particularly acute scrutiny and possible recrimination within the family, moral attributions are not confined to members of the kindred. Parents told us that adverse comments were not restricted to family members, but that their wider circle of friends and acquaintances had also suggested that they were in some way responsible for their child's problems. One mother recalled being asked directly by an acquaintance, 'What did you do?' This circle of implied blame extended in some cases to professionals involved in the care of the child, such as teachers and health visitors, who were said to have questioned their parenting skills. As one mother, whose child had been diagnosed with a syndrome that caused poor weight gain, described it: 'They [health visitors] accused me of taking food away from her' (Clinic 11, patient 1).

The attribution of personal agency and responsibility is not confined to the moral work of others. Self-blame is commonly expressed, and possible sources of responsibility are at least raised as possibilities in clinical consultations. Most commonly it was mothers who suggested that they were responsible for their child's problems. There were, however, instances where fathers sought reassurance from the clinical team, often volunteering specific events or behaviour in their past that they felt could be implicated. One father was concerned that environmental factors and aspects of his lifestyle in the past may have caused his child's condition. He had worked in a nuclear power station and 'took drugs'. His son had recently been diagnosed with polymicrogyria (Clinic 2, patient 1). The consultant geneticist reassured him that these factors were unlikely to be associated with the condition, clarifying the distinction that although his son had a genetic condition, it was not necessarily an inherited, familial condition. But his biographical search demonstrated the continuing significance of personal factors.

A wide range of biographical and interpersonal judgements informed the parents' feelings of guilt and the subsequent intense scrutiny they carried out of their own behaviour to identify the cause of their child's condition. The genetic nature of the referral itself often precipitated these feelings of guilt and added to their belief that the condition 'must have come from somewhere'. Parents, in particular mothers, expressed their own internal feelings of blame and guilt, which were exacerbated by the views of family members and wider social contacts. As a consequence, the moral and sentimental work of the clinic is often focused on the management of such feelings.

Absolving parents from blame

Parents who experience blame and self-blame receive scientific and moral absolution in the clinic. The clinical team routinely reassured parents who attended the genetics service that they were not to blame for their child's condition, and this was achieved in a number of ways. If the condition was identified as a *de novo* (spontaneous) mutation, then parents were reassured that they had not transmitted the condition to their child or caused it in some way through their lifestyle choices and behaviour. In those cases where the condition was a familial inherited condition, parents were also reassured that they were not to blame because they had no prior knowledge of their risk of transmitting this condition to their child, and also it presented only a risk of transmission rather than being an inevitability. In the following example a mother expresses her relief at her son's diagnosis. Even though the clinical team have been unable to diagnose a specific syndrome, they rule out a familial cause for the condition and this appears to alleviate her anxieties that she may be to blame:

CONSULTANT GENETICIST: Looking from a purely neurological point of view I can't see anything that's a problem.
[Specialist nurse takes child to the playroom.]
CONSULTANT GENETICIST: I've reviewed his notes and I don't think there's anything ... we've established a few things ...
MOTHER: I was so relieved when I got your letter [confirming the condition has nothing to do with her kidney disease during pregnancy]. I blamed myself all these years.

CONSULTANT GENETICIST: We can completely rule that out ... there's some type of genetic problem, likely to have occurred with him, there's nothing running through your family ...

(Clinic 1, patient 1)

Such explanations of aetiology do not mean that parental feelings of blame and responsibility disappear from their discourse. Parents still appeared to be searching for the reason it happened to them and to identify their role in causing their child's condition. In response to this, the clinic provided parents with high levels of reassurance in a number of ways.

The clinic functions as a site of reassurance for both parents and the clinical team. The pursuit of a genetic diagnosis provides parents with an extended time with an 'expert' on their child's condition. The child's development is monitored and assessed over an extended period during which a number of investigations are carried out, usually over a number of years. In turn, parents often reassured the clinical team about the benefits of attending the clinic, the development of the child and their ability to cope with their child's disabilities.

Parents often spoke of valuing the long-term support the clinic provided. Each consultation routinely included a detailed physical examination of the child by the same consultant and this typically involved a close examination of the child's body. These examinations were explicitly compared with, and judged against, previous assessments of the child's development and this is often an important source of reassurance for parents.

In the extract that follows, although the consultant says she is unsure whether she will be able to provide a definitive diagnosis of a named syndrome for their child, she can and does provide the parents with reassurance. The child's problems appear to be stable and are not deteriorating. She implies that this is good news for her long-term prognosis:

CONSULTANT GENETICIST: I'll also suggest some basic blood tests, though unlikely to be changes in the overall metabolism. We may or may not get an answer ... The important thing is her problems are static, they aren't getting worse ... This is in her favour
FATHER: I'm pleased it's static, we're dealing with what we've got.

(Clinic 3, patient 3)

The severity of the child's condition was often explicitly placed within the scale and severity of problems associated with the specific condition or syndrome. The consultant is a specialist in the field who is likely to have seen a similar case or diagnosed this rare syndrome before. The clinical team often reassured parents that their child had a mild form of the syndrome or was developing better than expected. Clinicians display their expertise by locating the child's condition within their own biographical frame of reference. Because they have seen a number of children with this rare condition, they are able to comment authoritatively on the child's likely future. In the following extract, the clinician says that, although the child's development is likely to be adversely affected by the syndrome, the extent of his developmental problems cannot be established through an MRI scan of his brain. However, she does add reassuringly that his development has been better than she would expect to see in children with this condition, explicitly listing his abilities and comparing him with other children she has seen with this syndrome:

CONSULTANT GENETICIST: Well, lots of seizures can impair development whatever his learning potential is. It's difficult to know, we can't really judge that from his MRI. His is milder than other forms of pachygyria. He's already doing more that I'd expect, sitting up, babbling, looking at the book … He's milder, he's lovely, he's interactive and a lovely boy, so it might be in his case intensive input could make a difference. I've seen a lot of children who I couldn't recommend.

(Clinic 2, patient 1)

The clinic is also a site for mutual reassurance. As well as receiving reassurance during clinical consultations, parents often reassured the clinical team about the benefits of attending the clinic, the development of their child and their ability to cope with their child's disabilities. For example, in the next extract, during the initial taking of a history by the consultant, this mother reassures her that in general her child is doing well despite the underlying discussion of the severe abnormalities and associated health problems this child has:

CONSULTANT GENETICIST: So really her development is fine?
MOTHER: Yes.
[Discussion of specific ear and feeding problems.]
CONSULTANT GENETICIST: Any other comments about her health generally?
MOTHER: She's doing really well.

(Clinic 7, patient 1)

Parents provided reassurance not only that they were coping with their child's disabilities but also that their child was a vitally important part of their family and made a significant contribution to family life. In the next example, a mother makes it clear to the team that, despite her son's severe developmental delay, she has no concerns or worries about him. She describes his ability to communicate, his sociability, the fact he has many friends, and that he has a good relationship with his sister. She concludes by saying:

MOTHER: We were talking about other things this morning. He's a lovely child, he's happy and healthy. It's got to the point when we'd like to know what's caused it. Some people are more intelligent than others.

I'll be happy if he's happy, if he gets a little job or stays with us for the rest of his life.

(Clinic 6, patient 2)

Parents provided this reassurance not only about the development and progress their child was making, but also in terms of the benefits they felt from attendance at the clinic itself, even where a diagnosis has not been made. During his clinical consultation one father said:

FATHER: Don't think that by finding no syndrome it's a problem. I see lots of kids where when you ask the parents and they don't know, but at least you've worked out that he hasn't got a lot of things that were worrying us.

(Clinic 5, patient 6)

In these contexts, parents provide performative displays of good family life, and enactments of good parenting. They affirm the essential moral worth of the child, and perform the normality of family relations (cf. Voysey 1975).

The sentimental repair work of the clinic

An important aspect of these clinical consultations was the work of repairing the perceptions of identity of the child and the family. Attendance at the clinic meant that parents were in an environment where their child was routinely admired by the clinical team, rather than treated as a source of shame and stigma. This is in marked contrast to these families' experiences in the wider community. Several families reported a wide range of negative reactions to their child that they had found upsetting and stigmatising.

One mother reported that she had found adults staring at her child when she took him swimming because of the growth on his back, which was not visible when he was clothed. In another, poignant account of a child with *cri du chat* syndrome, the baby's wailing which is characteristic of the condition, and hence gives the syndrome its name, meant that her parents were unable to 'hide' her condition. They felt that people in their local community crossed the road rather than meet them when they were out with their child.

The children who attended this clinic had dysmorphic features of varying severity, some of which related to the face or head. Some 'abnormal' physical features may be perceived as giving rise to a spoiled appearance: for example, *craniostenosis* (an enlargement of the skull). Paradoxically, some equally 'abnormal' features can also be extremely attractive. There are, for instance, children with elfin features, triangular faces and small stature which may be a feature of Russell–Silver syndrome. It is perhaps easier for conventionally attractive features to be seized on for compliments in the clinic, but, irrespective of the apparent severity of their dysmorphic features, all these children were described in similarly sentimental terms.

During the initial physical examination of the child, where physical abnormalities associated with an underlying syndrome are explicitly being sought, the clinical consultants would discuss their physical features. Although this was in the context of identifying a dysmorphic condition, the consultants routinely described the child in terms of their physical attractiveness. For example, a young boy with suspected Russell-Silver syndrome (the main features of which are small stature, asymmetry of limbs, a short and/or curved fifth finger and small triangular faces) is described as '*gorgeous*' and '*a little charmer*'; a little girl at risk of being affected with inherited cardiomyopathy (a disease of the heart muscle that can lead to sudden death) is a '*gorgeous little girl*', and a child with 22Q (associated with a deletion of the long arm of chromosome 22, this syndrome has variable dysmorphic features consisting of a round face, almond-shaped palpebral fissures, bulbous nose, malformed ears, hypotonia, short stature, learning disabilities, and other anomalies) is '*very sweet*'. The clinical team often explicitly described the child's features to parents in a positive way, using adjectives such as '*pretty*', '*handsome*' and '*gorgeous*'.

This extended to the examination of some children with severe physical abnormalities. In the example below, this young child has Goldenhar syndrome (*hemifacial microsomia*), his features are clearly asymmetric, and he has dysplastic ears (low and set back), large auricular tags (skin tags near the ear), *epibulbar dermoid* (ophthalmology problems) and mild facial weakness on his right side. The consultant concludes her examination by declaring that he is '*gorgeous*'. She appears to play down the severity of his abnormalities even in the face of parental insistence that his physical malformations are severe:

CONSULTANT GENETICIST: His asymmetry is not that marked.
MOTHER: The position of his ears is quite different.
CONSULTANT GENETICIST: [To the child, holding his head in her hands] You don't look too bad at all, in fact gorgeous!

(Clinic 4, patient 1)

Normal appearances – families and children

The clinical team performed the repair work of normalising families within the consultations. A wide range of behavioural characteristics displayed by children that were likely to be interpreted in other formal settings as problematic or disruptive were actively accepted and celebrated in the clinic. This was often in contrast to the families' experiences in the wider community, as they commonly reported during the interviews. For example, obstructive or noisy behaviour disrupting the clinic was never commented on by clinicians as a problem to be managed. It was not suggested that the child should be controlled or restrained by the parents. Instead, responses to such behaviour were universally positive. Children were described as '*mischievous*' and '*lively*' and to be enjoyed. The clinical team reinforced such behaviour as important signs of being a 'normal' child.

For example, during one consultation (Clinic 9, patient 1) the little boy was extremely disruptive and noisy, shouting, emptying a large metal waste bin, repeatedly trying to open the door and leave, opening cupboards and riding his tricycle round the room. The clinical team only intervened when there were concerns about his safety. During the relaxed and friendly consultation, his behaviour was celebrated and actively enjoyed by the team.

The clinical team used a number of devices to achieve this repair work. They commonly compared the child's behaviour with that experienced by 'normal' families, the clinician's own family, or commented on the universal nature of problems faced by parents. In the case below, the consultant reassures the mother that some of her child's behavioural problems are 'normal', adding that there are similar problems with the children in her own family:

MOTHER: Getting to sleep is a problem [she describes how difficult it is to get him to bed; she has to stay in the room with him until he is asleep, and when he stays with his grandmother he is allowed to sleep in her bed with her].

CONSULTANT GENETICIST: On the one hand he doesn't like to be on his own, but he also likes to have a grip on you.

MOTHER: I'm starting to limit how long I stay up there.

CONSULTANT GENETICIST: I know it's difficult with all children. I know in my family it's not much different.

(Clinic 1, patient 1)

Despite often severe developmental delay, or the presence of abnormalities, the clinical team frequently and explicitly categorised the children with other 'normal' children, emphasising their similarity. In one consultation, in the face of pressure from other professionals – in this case teachers at his nursery, who had suggested that the child's dribbling is abnormally severe – the specialist nurse reassured the anxious parents that this was within normal levels. As a former home visitor, the nurse described how he had seen many children with similar levels of dribbling, and suggested a simple treatment for the rash this causes.

The clinical team routinely reassured parents that they were doing the best for their child and praised them for being 'good parents'. In one example, the clinical team see a four-year-old boy with severe developmental delay. He has been attending the clinic for a number of years and, although a large number of investigations have been carried out, there is no diagnosis. He is attending the clinic because there is a suggestion that he may have Noonan syndrome. Noonan syndrome is associated with short stature, webbing of the neck, ear abnormalities, low posterior hairline and mild learning disabilities. The consultant paediatrician attending the consultation adds that he is 'a lovely little boy' and praises the parents for their child's lack of the behavioural difficulties often associated with his spectrum of problems. He says to the mother, 'He's one of these unusual children with developmental problems but no behavioural problems; that, I suspect, is a testament to you' (Clinic 5, patient 1).

The clinical team also stress normal parenting by acknowledging that the parents are the 'experts' who are best placed to judge their child's needs. They encourage a child-focused and common-sense approach to caring for these children, emphasising that the parents have the day-to-day experience of looking after their child.

The moral work of the clinic

Although the work of assembling a diagnosis is an important function of the clinic (Featherstone *et al.* 2005), other work is carried out within this setting that appears to have a significant function for families. Rather than the inability to provide parents with a definitive diagnosis resulting in a potential 'failure' of the clinic, the lengthy process of attending the clinic over a number of years in the search for a diagnosis, in itself, appears to provide parents with a number of benefits. An important function of the clinic is the moral and sentimental work it carries out.

The birth of a child with developmental problems can give rise to a culture of blame, affecting the views not only of the parents themselves who question their lifestyle and health behaviours, but also those among members of the wider family. Referral to the genetics clinic, its association with inherited 'familial' conditions, and the subsequent investigations of their child and their family (such as the examination of the family tree or 'pedigree') in the process of diagnosing a genetic syndrome, meant that parents were often concerned that they had been the cause of the disorder. In effect, this meant that parents scrutinised themselves and their wider family for an associated disorder or for signs that they could have contributed to or caused their child's condition in some way. This also extended to their own behaviour and lifestyle to try to make sense of what had happened. In addition, parents reported that they in turn were scrutinised by other members of their family for signs that they may have caused the condition, a practice we have described elsewhere as 'mutual surveillance' (Featherstone *et al.* 2006). This led to complex beliefs about the aetiology of their child's condition and understandings of inheritance and causation. Thus, because a genetic diagnosis has the potential to identify the origins of the condition and (if familial) the potential route of inheritance, the clinic also provides the opportunity for the attribution of blame and responsibility for transmission.

Whilst in many ways responsible for causing these concerns, the clinic provided parents with a discreet and professional space in which to confide their fears about their role in causing their child's condition. Within this setting, parents often confessed to acts or omissions, particularly connected to their lifestyle, that they felt may be associated with the cause of their child's problems in some way. Parents often appeared to be highly anxious when they attended the clinic, particularly if this was their first appointment. During this initial consultation, a detailed history was routinely taken and this was often the point at which parents chose to inform the clinician about behaviour or events that they believe may have contributed to or caused their child's problems. The style of such disclosures often took the form of a confessional, their speech was often hesitant, and they appeared to be relieved once they had unburdened themselves of what had been secret fears. The finding of a genetic cause meant that parents could address these feelings of guilt and responsibility and this is consistent with the findings of earlier studies (Carmichael *et al.* 1999; Collins *et al.* 2001; Barr and Millar 2003). Thus, attending the clinic allowed parents to discuss their often complex feelings of guilt.

Armstrong *et al.* (1998) suggest that clients (whose clinic transcripts they studied) who offered such non-genetic explanations – such as diet or medication – in response to their diagnosis were doing so as a diversionary tactic, in order to evade the reality of a genetic cause for the condition. However, our research suggests that parental scrutiny of their behaviour and lifestyle in the light of a genetic diagnosis is a way for them and their families to make sense of the condition. These families are not avoiding the genetic nature of their child's condition but are seeking ways to understand why this has happened to their child. Personal responsibility and genetic fate are interwoven in parents' accounts and their search for explanations.

As we have seen, the clinic functions as an important site of reassurance for both parents and the clinical team. The pursuit of a genetic diagnosis often took a number of years, and in some cases never led to an explicit diagnosis of a named syndrome, although in such cases the clinic was usually able to provide parents with the likely cause of their child's problems. Although the provision of a diagnosis was important for the majority of parents, their connection with the clinic often did not stop at that point. Parents felt that they had an ongoing relationship with the clinical genetics team, which was based upon factors other than that of risk assessment. They continued to use the clinic as an important point of reference to monitor their child's development, and they valued the regular progress reviews. They all felt that, even if they stopped attending, they were in no doubt that they could contact the clinic if they had concerns about their child at some point in the future. Bernhardt *et al.* (2000) similarly found that families valued the ongoing contact with the clinic, particularly being able to have their child's development assessed by someone regarded as an expert in the field.

More recently, Barr and Millar (2003) have reported that the genetics service attended by the families they interviewed did not provide ongoing support once a diagnosis had been provided, which suggests that there is some variation in the organisation of clinical services. While previous studies have argued for ongoing contact between the genetics service and parents of children with inherited conditions, our research shows that a genetics service that is able to sustain a relationship over a period of time, with contact not limited to a diagnostic and future risk assessment role, can play a wider role in supporting parents.

The clinical management of children has been a major theme in the sociological analysis of medical institutions and the attribution of identities (cf. Bluebond-Langner 1978). The intervention of medical services and members of other caring professions in the lives of children and their families gives rise to delicate moral and identity work. The identity and value of the child may be under threat, and may be re-affirmed through interactive face-to-face work; the moral worth of parents may also be a topic of identity work in both professionalised and everyday encounters (cf. Voysey 1975). As Davis and Strong (1976) point out, the value and attractiveness of children is repeatedly affirmed in the context of paediatric encounters (Davis and Strong 1976). The maxim 'aren't children wonderful' (maintained irrespective of their actual performance) captures the taken-for-granted value of children. Likewise, Voysey's analysis of parental accounts in families with a child with disabilities demonstrates vividly the moral work of accounting for 'normal' parenting and 'normal' family life in the face of others' presumptions of family difficulty (Voysey 1975). Such work has salience for the work of the genetics clinic, particularly within the specialism of dysmorphology. As we have seen, the moral order of normal family life and the maintenance of personal identities is a co-production between parents and members of the clinical team. This co-production of identities is achieved against a backdrop of implied or actual threats to parents' identity, and to that of the dysmorphic child. Possible attributions of blame, responsibility and stigma are, in turn, enmeshed in the everyday theodicy of genetic medicine. Parents make sense of genetic conditions by incorporating registers of personal causation and responsibility in the impersonal frameworks of biological causation. Such interpretative framing is two-edged. On the one hand, it may help to render misfortune explicable. On the other hand, the insertion of personal causation has implications for personal blame and interpersonal recrimination.

Dysmorphia in children clearly throws into relief identity work in medical settings. First, dysmorphia gives rise to actual or potential threats to the attributed identity of the child, through the potentially stigmatising implications of spoiled appearance (Goffman 1968). Second, the fact that it is implicated in *genetic* medicine creates the potential for moral threats to the parents' and their families' identities. An important aspect of the clinical consultations observed in this study was the work of repairing the perceptions of identity of the child and the family. Many of the families reported a wide range of negative reactions to their child in the wider community (and in some cases by other professionals) that they found upsetting and stigmatising.

In most cases, these children had learning disabilities, and often had dysmorphic features of varying severity, some of which related to the face or head. Attendance at the clinic meant that parents were in an environment where their child was routinely admired by the clinical team, rather than treated as a potential source of shame and stigma. Irrespective of the apparent severity of their dysmorphic features, all these children were described in similarly sentimental terms. In addition, a wide range of behavioural characteristics displayed by children and likely to be interpreted in other formal settings as problematic or disruptive were actively accepted and enjoyed within the clinic.

This finding is interesting – it might be felt that the work of the dysmorphology clinic would contribute to parental feelings of stigma and shame. As we have documented elsewhere (Featherstone *et al.* 2005), within these clinics both the children and their families are scrutinised intensely. Children's bodies and faces are closely scrutinised for 'abnormalities', and are routinely photographed. Parents and other family members may also be examined physically, and a family history is routinely taken, which encourages the disclosure of stories of any other family members with physical abnormalities or learning disabilities.

The clinical team used a number of devices to achieve this repair work. They commonly compared the child's behaviour to that experienced by 'normal' families and even the clinician's own family, or by commenting on the universal nature of problems faced by parents. Despite often-severe developmental delay or abnormalities being present, the clinical team explicitly grouped these children with other 'normal' children, emphasising their sameness. Where families felt the stigma of having a child who is not completely normal which can be seen in external features or behavioural problems, the clinician redressed the balance by positively highlighting the child's abilities and providing assurance about their development.

This research suggests that ongoing contact with the genetics clinic serves to fill a wider role than simply that of providing a diagnosis. It is a role that parents value. Although obtaining a diagnosis can be very important to families, such contact beyond diagnosis can provide important support for the parents and may well be in direct contrast to the attitudes they encounter in other areas of their life.

Acknowledgements

The support of the Economic and Social Research Council (ESRC) is gratefully acknowledged. This work was part of the programme of the ESRC Centre for Economic and Social Aspects of Genomics (CESAGen). We would also like to thank all the families who took part, and Daniella Pilz, Angus Clarke, Linda Jones, Alan Cowe, Hayley Archer, Sarah Buston and Charlotte Riddick, for their contribution to the project.

References

Aase, J. M. (1990) *Diagnostic Dysmorphology*. New York: Plenum Medical.

Armstrong, D., Michie, S. and Marteau, T. (1998) 'Revealed identity: a study of the process of genetic counselling', *Social Science & Medicine*, 47 (11): 1653–8.

Barr, O. and Millar, R. (2003) 'Parents of children with intellectual disabilities: their expectations and experience of genetic counselling', *Journal of Applied Research in Intellectual Disabilities*, 16 (3): 189–204.

Bernhardt, B. A., Biesecker, B. B. and Mastromarino, C. L. (2000) 'Goals, benefits, and outcomes of genetic counselling: client and genetic counsellor assessment', *American Journal of Medical Genetics*, 94 (3): 189–97.

Biesecker, B. B. (2001) 'Goals of genetic counselling', *Clinical Genetics*, 60(5): 323–30.

Birenbaum, A. (1992) 'Courtesy stigma revisited', *Mental Retardation*, 30(5): 265–8.

Black, R. B., (1980) 'Parents' evaluations of genetic counselling', *Patient Counselling and Health Education*, 2 (3): 142–6.

Bluebond-Langner, M. (1978) *The Private Lives of Dying Children*. Princeton, NJ: Princeton University Press.

Brett, J. (2002) 'The experience of disability from the perspective of parents of children with profound impairment: is it time for an alternative model of disability?', *Disability and Society*, 17 (7): 825–43.

Britten N. (1995) 'Qualitative interviews in medical research', *British Medical Journal*, 311: 251-3.

Carlton-Ford, S., Miller, R., Nealeigh, N. and Sanchez, N. (1997) 'The effects of perceived stigma and psychological over-control on the behavioural problems of children with epilepsy', *Seizure: The Journal of the British Epilepsy Association*, 6 (5): 383–91.

Carmichael, B., Pembrey, M., Turner, G. and Barnicoat, A. (1999) 'Diagnosis of fragile-X syndrome: the experiences of parents', *Journal of Intellectual Disability Research*, 43 (1): 47–53.

Collins, V., Halliday, J., Kahler, S. and Williamson, R. (2001) 'Parents' experiences with genetic counseling after the birth of a baby with a genetic disorder: an exploratory study', *Journal of Genetic Counselling*, 10 (1): 53–72.

Davis A. (1982) *Children in Clinics*. London: Tavistock.

Davis, A. G. and Strong, P. M. (1976) 'Aren't children wonderful? A study of the allocation of identity in developmental assessment', in Stacey, M. (ed.), *The Sociology of the National Health Service*, Monograph 22. Keele: University of Keele.

Elwyn, G., Gray, J. and Iredale, R. (2000) 'Tensions in implementing the new genetics. General practitioners in south Wales are unconvinced of their role in genetics services', *British Medical Journal*, 321 (7255): 240–1.

Evers-Kiebooms, G. and Van Den Berghe, H. (1979) 'Impact of genetic counselling: A review of published follow-up studies', *Clinical Genetics*, 15 (6): 465–74.

Featherstone, K., Atkinson P. A., Bharadwaj, A. and Clarke, A. J. (2006) *Risky Relations: family, kinship and the new genetics*. Oxford: Berg.

Featherstone, K., Latimer, J., Atkinson, P., Clarke, A. and Pilz, D. (2005) 'Dysmorphology and the spectacle of the clinic', *Sociology of Health and Illness*, 27 (5): 551–74.

Goffman, E. (1968) [1963] *Stigma: notes on the management of spoiled identity*. Harmondsworth: Penguin Books.

Gray, D. E. (2002) '"Everybody just freezes. Everybody is just embarrassed": felt and enacted stigma among parents of children with high functioning autism', *Sociology of Health & Illness*, 24 (6): 734–49.

Green, S. E. (2003) '"What do you mean 'what's wrong with her?'": stigma and the lives of families of children with disabilities', *Social Science & Medicine*, 57 (8): 1361–74.

Hallowell, N. and Murton, F. (1998) 'The value of written summaries of genetic consultations', *Patient Education and Counselling*, 35 (1): 27–34.

Hanus, S. H., Bernstein, N. R., and Kapp, K. A. (1981) 'Immigrants into society. Children with craniofacial anomalies', *Clinical pediatrics*, 20 (1): 37–41.

Harper, P. S. (1998) *Practical Genetic Counselling*, 5th edn. Oxford: Butterworth Heinemann.

Jones, K. L. (1997) *Smith's Recognizable Patterns of Human Malformation*, 5th edn. Philadelphia, PA: W. B. Saunders.

Kessler, S. (1997) 'Psychological aspects of genetic counselling: IX. Teaching and Counselling', *Journal of Genetic Counselling*, 6: 287–95.

Latner, J. D. and Stunkard, A. J. (2003) 'Getting worse: the stigmatization of obese children', *Obesity Research*, 11 (3): 452–6.

McConkie-Rosell, A. and Sullivan, J. A. (1999) 'Genetic counselling-stress, coping and the empowerment perspective', *Journal of Genetic Counselling*, 8 (6): 345–57.

McKeever, P. and Miller, K. (2004) 'Mothering children who have disabilities: a Bourdieusian interpretation of maternal practices', *Social Science and Medicine*, 59 (6): 1177–91.

Mays, N. and Pope, C. (1995) 'Rigour and qualitative research', *British Medical Journal*, 311: 109-12.

Michie, S., Axworthy, D., Weinman, J. and Marteau, T. (1996) 'Genetic counselling: Predicting patient outcomes', *Psychology & Health*, 11 (6): 797–809.

Michie, S., McDonald, V. and Marteau, T. M. (1997) 'Genetic counselling: information given, recall and satisfaction', *Patient Education and Counselling*, 32, 101–6.

Michie, S., Marteau, T. M. and Bobrow, M. (1994) 'Genetic counselling: the psychological impact of meeting patients' expectations', *Journal of Medical Genetics*, 34 (3): 237–41.

Norvilitis, J. M., Scime, M. and Lee, J. S. (2002) 'Courtesy stigma in mothers of children with attention-deficit/hyperactivity disorder: a preliminary investigation', *Journal of Attention Disorders*, 6 (2): 61–8

Pilnick, A. and Dingwall, R. (2001) 'Research directions in genetic counselling: a review of the literature', *Patient Education and Counselling*, 44: 95–105.

Prussing, E., Sobo, E. J., Walker, E. and Kurtin, P. S. (2005) 'Between "desperation" and disability rights: A narrative analysis of complementary/alternative medicine use by parents for children with Down syndrome', *Social Science & Medicine*, 60 (3): 587–98.

Segal, R., Mandich, A., Polatajko, H. and Cook, J. V. (2002) 'Stigma and its management: a pilot study of parental perceptions of the experiences of children with developmental coordination disorder', *The American Journal of Occupational Therapy: official publication of the American Occupational Therapy Association*, 56 (4): 422–8.

Shiloh, S., Avdor, O. and Goodman R. M. (1990) 'Satisfaction with genetic counselling: dimensions and measurement', *American Journal of Medical Genetics*, 37 (4): 522–9.

Skirton, H. (2001) 'The client's perspective of genetic counselling: a grounded theory study', *Journal of Genetic Counselling*, 10 (4): 311–29.

Somer, M., Mustonen, H. and Norio, R. (1988) 'Evaluation of genetic counselling: recall of information, post-counselling reproduction, and attitude of the counsellees', *Clinical Genetics*, 34 (6): 352–65.

Strong, P. M. (1979) *The Ceremonial Order of the Clinic: parents, doctors and medical bureaucracies*. London: Routledge and Kegan Paul.

Strong P. and Davis A. (1978) 'Who's who in paediatric encounters: morality, expertise, and the generation of identity and action in medical settings', in A. Davis (ed.), *Relationships Between Doctors and Patients*. Farnborough: Teakfield.

van Riper, M., Pridham, K. and Ryff, C. (1992) 'Symbolic interactionism: a perspective for understanding parent–nurse interactions following the birth of a child with Down syndrome', *Maternal-child Nursing Journal*, 20 (3–4): 21–39.

Voysey, M. (1975) *A Constant Burden*. London: Routledge and Kegan Paul.

Wang, C., Gonzalez, R. and Merajver, S. D. (2004) 'Assessment of genetic testing and related counselling services: current research and future directions', *Social Science & Medicine*, 58 (7): 1427–42.

8 Medical classification and the experience of genetic haemochromatosis

Aditya Bharadwaj, Paul Atkinson and Angus Clarke

Introduction

DNA-based biomedical technologies create the possibility for new topographies of physiology and pathology. Based on biomedical science at the molecular level, these technologies are increasingly mapping disease in clinics and laboratories through genetically informed talk and work (Atkinson *et al.* 2001; Bharadwaj 2002). Genetic medicine is increasingly developing new biological and clinical categories, contributing to what Keating and Cambrosio (2003) refer to as 'biomedical platforms' that comprise new configurations of knowledge derived from the intersections of laboratory science and clinical practice. New genetic technologies create the possibility of new biomedical knowledge and the transformation of clinical entities. They also give rise to new definitions of health and illness. The identification of genetic risks or genetic susceptibility to one or more of a range of genetically-transmitted diseases can create new ambiguous categories of person who are neither perfectly healthy nor clinically sick, but 'at risk'. The opportunity to screen populations for a growing number of conditions will create ever greater numbers of individuals who find themselves in such a position. While risk is not confined to genetic constitutions, and there are many risks defined by lifestyle and other circumstances, the estimation of genetic risk is a new technology of medical classification. It gives rise to the possibility of what we have called elsewhere the 'genetic iceberg' of susceptibility and potential anxiety (Bharadwaj *et al.* 2006; Bharadwaj 2002). There is, therefore, an intimate relationship between the changing boundaries and classifications of genetic disease and the shifting categories of patienthood and personal identity.

Genetic haemochromatosis (GH) is one disease that has acquired new clinical and scientific significance since the discovery of the *HFE* gene in 1996 (Beutler *et al.* 2002). Haemochromatosis is a genetic disorder causing the body to absorb an excessive amount of iron from the diet (Bothwell and MacPhail 1998). The excess iron is subsequently deposited in multiple organs, especially the liver, pancreas, heart, endocrine glands and joints. Excessive quantities of iron trigger progressive liver disease and may also cause serious damage in other organs and body parts (Niederau *et al.* 1996; Bothwell and MacPhail 1998). The susceptibility to absorb excessive amounts of iron is usually associated with homozygosity for a particular mutation of the *HFE* gene. Since its discovery in 1996, this mutation (the *C282Y* mutation of the *HFE* gene) has been identified as the underlying cause of haemochromatosis in over 80 per cent of the patients (Beutler *et al.* 2002). It is estimated that in Europe, Australia and the USA 60–100 per cent of patients with genetic haemochromatosis are homozygous for this mutation (Worwood 1999). In Britain 1 in 200 people are susceptible homozygotes (i.e. they carry two copies of the mutation); the proportion who develop clinical haemochromatosis is small but not clearly defined. Therefore, while it is possible to screen individuals with the view to predicting their personal susceptibility to developing the condition, such risk prognostications are often tentative. A positive test result demonstrating this double dose of the mutant gene identifies an otherwise healthy individual only as *susceptible* to the development of the disorder. A recent study in South Wales, the region of our own study, showed that only one per cent of adult GH homozygotes had a clinical diagnosis of iron overload (McCune *et al.* 2002).

There is as yet no firm clinical basis for the prediction of when and how a healthy susceptible individual develops frank disease or overt iron overload, although it is becoming clear that variation at other genetic loci as well as environmental factors including diet are all relevant. Measurement of body iron stores serves as a proxy indicator – a very imperfect predictor – of future disease onset. This leaves clinicians and scientists still grappling with the multifactorial complexities underlying the condition. Conversely, the clinical diagnosis of haemochromatosis is by no means straightforward. Symptoms of iron overload are often diffuse, including lassitude and signs of impaired liver function. Primary health practitioners may readily attribute them to a variety of underlying causes other than haemochromatosis. If identified, the condition can normally be managed through regular bleeding, which depletes the body's excess iron, and the condition is eminently treatable (Niederau *et al.* 1996). If it remains undiagnosed, then serious organ damage can result. (See McDonnell *et al.* 1999 for a survey of 2,851 patients' experiences and symptoms.) In the current state of genetic knowledge and clinical practice, therefore, it is possible to identify individuals who have an inherited susceptibility to GH, but with only restricted prediction of disease onset, and it is equally possible to identify GH patients whose condition has been misdiagnosed or diagnosed late, and whose genetic status is only confirmed retrospectively. While it is not the main focus of this chapter, it should be noted, therefore, that the uncertainties surrounding clinical diagnosis make it very difficult to assess the penetrance of the gene with any degree of precision.

Here we document how haemochromatosis and its clinical management are experienced and understood by a series of individuals who have been identified as affected by the condition. We examine the lay phenomenology of haemochromatosis: how affected patients make sense of the condition. We argue that individuals with GH may attempt actively to contribute to the production and narration of the condition by critically engaging with the clinical nosography. This creates what Waldby (2000: 466) has called 'multiple ontologies of bodies, disease and medically constituted subjectivities' amongst patients. Haemochromatosis patients are, in other words, engaged in making sense of the disease and seek actively to challenge and extend the boundaries of expert classifications and boundaries. Patients explore the interpretative space that is created by the relatively uncertain nature of the clinical diagnosis of haemochromatosis. Many of the affected individuals with frank symptoms of the condition report that they experienced difficulty in having their illness acknowledged and validated by medical practitioners. As a consequence, the disciplinary practices of the clinic – medicalisation, normalisation and objectification – are *sought* by patients in pursuit of clinical validation of their symptomatic manifestations of GH.

Recent accounts of the construction of genetic disease include analyses of the 'expansion' of diagnostic categories and clinical entities. In particular, Kerr (2000, 2004) and Hedgecoe (2003, 2004), examining the 'geneticisation' of cystic fibrosis (CF), have discussed the process whereby genetic medicine may extend the boundaries of the disease to include new clinical phenomena within its ambit: in the case of CF the boundary may be expanded to capture one variety of male infertility. The identification of genetic bases for a widening number of conditions can shift the boundaries of diseases and syndromes previously identified primarily on clinical grounds. The analytic value of the notion of 'geneticisation' in this context has been contested. It is clear that, on the basis of detailed explorations of the practice of contemporary genetic medicine, there is not a simple, reductionist process whereby genetic conditions become 'fixed' as a consequence of diagnostic genetic investigations. While susceptibility to GH can be identified in terms of genetic categories, new genetic technologies do not determine the classification and phenomenology of the condition. We should, therefore, be cautious (at best) of endorsing general claims as to the geneticisation of contemporary medicine, or that new genetic technologies necessarily determine professional and lay conceptions of clinical entities. It is certainly premature to extrapolate from specific cases to make general claims about the geneticisation of health and medicine *in toto*. These remain empirical issues. We are thus sceptical about the sort of claims made by Finkler (2000), or Haraway (1990), who suggest – from very different perspectives – that contemporary genetic technologies necessarily transform the nature of medical knowledge and lead inexorably to a geneticisation of medicine or the geneticisation of identity.

It would, therefore, be inaccurate to account for the consequences of new genetic medicine in terms of a simple, unilinear process whereby genetic science progressively furnishes unequivocal grounds for determining the boundaries and diagnostic criteria of clinical entities. It is not only clinical geneticists and clinical scientists who can find themselves expanding or contesting the boundaries of disease classifications and criteria, however. Patients who find themselves experiencing a genetic disorder may also be engaged in exploring and contesting such boundaries. In this chapter we describe how patients with genetic haemochromatosis (GH) may seek to expand the condition to incorporate their everyday symptoms for inclusion within the nosography of the disease. When professional classifications are uncertain and shifting, lay nosographies of genetic disorders are implicated in the process of diagnostic inference. It is not necessary to invoke the notion of lay expertise (cf. Arksey 1994; Busby, Williams and Rogers 1997; Epstein 1995; Sarangi 2001) to recognise that the mundane phenomenology of illness can have considerable significance for patients and professionals in mapping clinical illness. As Prior's review highlights, claims concerning expertise on the part of patients, activists and other lay actors can readily mask significant differences in the *forms* of knowledge between lay persons and professional practitioners (Prior 2003). Lay actors may undoubtedly become knowledgeable about restricted and specific phenomena, often on the basis of personal experience. But that does not mean that we can unequivocally assign them expert knowledge without emptying the latter of any analytic force.

In approaching patients' accounts of their own conditions we do not assume *a priori* a high degree of symmetry between the contents of patients' and professionals' knowledge. We do not assume that patients should necessarily be regarded as lay 'experts' on their own conditions, nor that one should equate their practical interests with the knowledge of professionals. There are qualitative differences between the two. Patients can undoubtedly become highly proficient in recognising illness, symptoms and changes in physical status in their own bodies and in those of family members and other intimates. When they have a specific illness they can also become adept at describing, tracing and monitoring its physical and emotional effects. They become, in other words, practical phenomenologists primarily in illnesses that are their own or that they socially share. The illness can become a central feature of their own lifeworld. The particularities of the patient's own condition may well present themselves differently from the generic categories of the professional practitioner's knowledge. The professional is expert not in the particularities of the case but in the general categories of medical knowledge. Her or his knowledge is not grounded in the practical phenomenology of the self and the body, but in the theoretical knowledge of ideal-typical disease categories (cf. Mishler 1984). There are, however, some key aspects in which the interests of the lay and professional observer coincide. Both are engaged in the attempt to identify the appropriate characteristics, criteria and boundaries of diagnostic and pathological classifications. The patient seeks to establish one or both of two issues: Are all my symptoms explained by the disease I have been diagnosed with? Will the medical profession accept my own descriptions of my symptoms and grant them legitimacy within the clinical description of my condition? The medical practitioner is also concerned with establishing the patient's condition (symptoms, signs, family history, laboratory results) as a 'case' of an ideal-typical illness category. Both, therefore, have interests in tracing the boundaries between the normal and the pathological, and in mapping the categories of 'normal' disease entities. As we shall discuss more fully below, the epistemological problem of the boundaries of the normal and the pathological are not confined to the realm of the philosopher (e.g. Canguilhem 1989): they are also practical issues for lay and professional actors alike. Moreover, both have interests in identifying what is to count as 'normal' pathology, as opposed to idiopathic variations or coincidental symptoms.

Haemochromatosis: the research

Our discussion is derived from research on individuals identified as either affected by, or at risk of, iron overload from genetic haemochromatosis in three regional centres in England and Wales (Cardiff, Cambridge and Southampton). The larger research project compares those individuals presenting symptoms of the disease as a result of the *HFE* mutation with healthy blood donors shown to be potentially susceptible to the condition, through carrying two copies of the C282Y mutation, but as yet having no clinical manifestations of the disease. The blood donors had previously been identified through genetic testing carried out as part of a separate research investigation of the natural history of the condition in South Wales. Blood donors had been screened, and on the basis of such screening a number were identified as homozygous, and therefore susceptible to developing clinical haemochromatosis at some time in the future. The broader aim of our research is to contribute to the ongoing debate on the desirability of population screening for genetic diseases (Clarke 1995; Harper and Clarke 1995; Davis 1998; Burke *et al.* 1998; Allen and Williamson 1999; Seamark 2000; Allen and Williamson 2000; Evans *et al.* 2001; Williamson *et al.* 2001; Beutler *et al.* 2002). The identification of haemochromatosis susceptibility or risk in the blood-donors study provides one possible research model for wider programmes of population genetic screening and their personal consequences. We compared the experiences of asymptomatic individuals who were 'at risk' with the experience of patients with clinical haemochromatosis.

The research is a multidisciplinary collaboration between social scientists, clinical geneticists and haematologists. Through this collaboration the research has established how to dovetail the social and clinical research in order to avoid an unreasonable research burden on the enrolled participants and to optimise the cross-disciplinary sharing of research between the clinical and social research projects.

Fieldwork involved in-depth interviews with twenty asymptomatic blood donors in South Wales, twenty-five symptomatic individuals from three different clinics in Wales and England, and nine members of The Haemochromatosis Society. Access to informants in South Wales was obtained through a larger clinical study involving blood donors (Jackson *et al.* 2001). A call for research participation published in the Haemochromatosis Society newsletter enabled the recruitment of informants from among the membership. Individual patients were approached in the other clinics, where they were given additional information on the project by the researcher. The majority of the interviews were conducted at the informant's home, with the exception of the Southampton sample, where a separate room was made available for interviews within the clinic. Through in-depth interviews with clinicians and other experts we have also collected expert opinion concerning the diagnosis of GH and the potential value and implications of adult-population screening. Clinics were observed in the three different haematology services. The research has yielded accounts from both healthy asymptomatic individuals and individuals with clinical manifestations of haemochromatosis (some severely ill) as well as clinicians, haematologists, geneticists, and scientists engaged in routine laboratory work. All interviews were transcribed and anonymised for subsequent analysis. The analyses focused mainly on the informants' accounts of the impact of diagnosis, and their personal constructions of susceptibility; their assessments of healthcare and support; and their personal experience of living with the disease. The accounts of experts and medical staff were analysed to ascertain and explore issues of uncertainty concerning the diagnosis and prognosis of the condition; their narrative devices to explain the meaning of risk and susceptibility in the context of genetic conditions like haemochromatosis; and their views on the likely value of future population screening.

For the purposes of this discussion we draw only on accounts of people living with haemochromatosis and its most notable pathological manifestations: we do not here include any accounts from the healthy, but mutation-positive, blood donors. The examples come from semi-structured interviews with the sixteen patients, who are drawn from a wide range of differing backgrounds such as retired nurse, builder, engineer, self-employed and homemaker. All informants are married and those in employment have their incomes pooled with their partners'. The class position of the interviewees ranges from unemployed working-class to middle-class homemakers. The interviewees' ages range from 45 to 67. Pseudonyms are used throughout. The research with this series of haemochromatosis sufferers was conducted through extended, semi-structured interviews, in which were explored their personal experiences of the condition, the processes whereby they had sought and received a clinical diagnosis, and their understandings of the disease and its aetiology. The interviews were tape-recorded and transcribed verbatim. We have reported them with minimal stylistic or grammatical changes.

Haemochromatosis: a nosography under construction

The definitive nosography of haemochromatosis is as yet unavailable; indeed, a systematic description of the disease is proving difficult to generate. In order to identify individuals with the genetic susceptibility and to predict their progression from health through iron accumulation to evidence of toxicity in the form of the signs and symptoms of haemochromatosis would require a large-scale, longitudinal study following a birth cohort that had been tested for the *C282Y* mutation. While such gold-standard evidence is not available, specialists have to manage with what has been found in published studies of affected individuals and families. Early clinical and family descriptions of haemochromatosis, including those by Debre *et al.* (1958) and Bothwell *et al.* (1959), suggested that haemochromatosis was often autosomal dominant in inheritance. It was not until the work published by Saddi and Feingold (1974), Simon *et al.* (1977) and finally Bassett *et al.* (1982) that it was safe to conclude that it is an autosomal recessive susceptibility. In other words, an individual who inherits two copies of the mutation is susceptible to developing the condition. But penetrance is partial: the presence and severity of the clinical condition cannot be predicted with certainty from the genotype. Untreated haemochromatosis can lead to serious illness, with significant damage to affected organs. If identified at a sufficiently early stage, however, its clinical management is usually straightforward: iron overload is depleted through regular bleeding (phlebotomy). Because the onset of the clinical condition is insidious, however, it can readily progress unrecognised, with symptoms attributed to a variety of other underlying causes.

Clinical studies have identified the principal features of the disease as: arthritis and joint pain, cirrhosis – and sometimes carcinoma – of the liver, bronzing of the skin, pancreatic failure and diabetes, other endocrine problems, and sexual dysfunction, hair loss, headaches, depression and fatigue. While these features of the disease have long been acknowledged in the clinically accepted description of haemochromatosis, individuals participating in our own research embodied greatly divergent symptoms – some of which find no place in the clinical description of haemochromatosis. When patients claim that such symptoms are caused by their haemochromatosis, they report resistance from professionals. Such apparent reluctance on the part of medical practitioners may stem partly from a general scepticism, based on the assumption that association indicates no more than mere (perhaps repeated) coincidence. Our interviews with expert practitioners suggest that reluctance is also motivated by the assumption that the description of a clinical entity involves powerful causal claims – aetiological, anatomical or histopathological, clinical or prognostic (Keating and Cambrosio 2003, 106). It may be difficult for a practitioner to accede to a patient's suggestion that a given symptom is a result of haemochromatosis if such a symptom is not a part of the standardised description. Patients' own descriptions of their symptoms and their own configurations of their conditions can readily be at odds with the normal typifications of clinical medicine. Their personal nosography can thus present an implicit challenge to the classificatory system of practitioners' nosographies.

The possibility of such differences, or even contestations, derives in part from the somewhat diffuse character of the condition, and from the insidious nature of its manifestation. The identification of clinical, symptomatic haemochromatosis is often far from straightforward. As the following extract from our interview with Patrick suggests, symptoms can be diffuse, and do not necessarily conform to a readily identifiable pattern.

P: I actually felt like shit. I didn't want to get out of bed, I didn't want to go anywhere, I didn't want to see anyone, speak to any, I just didn't want to do anything. I just, and I couldn't explain why. And when I went to see my doctor he would say to me 'How are you?' I says 'I don't know,' I says 'I feel dreadful,' I says 'But I can't sort of pinpoint any specific thing about what was happening to me.' And then like my hands started to swell up, my knees swelled up, my ankles swelled up, I became, my wrists began to get sore, I was finding it difficult to hold a pen, anything small and thin I was having real problems like holding. I mean I had problems holding plates and all the other things as well but up until when I was diagnosed I couldn't understand what was happening to me. And of course all my mates sort of like thought oh he's a bloody hypochondriac you know he's always ill ... But it's a very, very weird like illness to have if you like because I've now got other problems with hormones. I have to have injections every month because my testosterone levels were very, very low, I was losing like a lot of body hair, I mean I virtually lost all the hair on my arms and my legs and like parts of my chest and like down my stomach because I was quite a hairy person. ... So I saw my endocrine doctor who's also my diabetic doctor and he sort of like did tests on things and I've got something that my pituitary gland doesn't work a hundred percent the way it should, but it's not at a level where I need to have treatment for it, it's still functioning just enough. But I'm waiting for a decision from the hospital about the growth hormone.

AB: Are they relating this to haemochromatosis?

P: Yeah

AB: All of this?

P: They reckon that all of this is down to the haemochromatosis. They actually think that the diabetes was down to the haemochromatosis as well although at the time we didn't know it ...

Early detection of Patrick's condition would have permitted the earlier commencement of preventive phlebotomy – that would have allowed clinicians to monitor his iron levels, and would have prevented iron accumulation in the blood, joints and other organs. Like many patients, the main difficulty Patrick had had to face was the silent build-up of iron stores with no obvious symptoms and the subsequent delay in diagnosis. Once diagnosed, however, his symptoms and the attendant manifestations of the disease were taken to conform to the established clinical nosography of genetic haemochromatosis. Once his symptoms were identified, in other words, Patrick was clinically allocated to the typification of a 'normal' disease entity. Normal illness classifications reside in the capacity of the clinician to apply her or his practical professional competence to fit a variety of symptoms to a clinical typification (cf Atkinson 1997: 173–81).

Diagnostic delays are recognised by patients and professionals as all too common. Mary Shaw, a 52-year-old swimming teacher, is a patient whose account was suffused with anger at the loss of crucial years because of her GP's perceived inability to diagnose her symptoms and arrange for a timely referral.

M: Oh yes. I mean it would've been very nice if somebody somewhere along the line probably two or three years beforehand had put it all together.

AB: Sure.

M: But it was only me that kept on and on and on saying you know this isn't right, that's not right there's got to be something that is causing all of this, but no one put it together. I mean even like early menopause, I was 42 or something, you know, everything, I had the lot but no one had put it together. And I really didn't find my GP very helpful at all.

AB: No? In what way?

M: Well since the day I've been diagnosed he's never even asked me how I am or how's it going or what's happening, not at all interested. Quite open, 'Oh I don't understand it really', and he just never asked me. And I find that really hard you know when I've been going to him for so long feeling so awful that you know he could've, I just, I feel he could've said 'I'm really sorry I didn't know about this but you know we've come up with something and you know maybe I should have picked it up and maybe I'll pick it up in the future', but nothing, just nothing.

AB: And do you find him particularly lacking in terms of understanding of haemochromatosis?

M: Oh he's got none at all.

AB: He doesn't have any?

M: No, no. I mean I have, I can't say I've changed GPs, I go to quite a large surgery and my way out of it was that I said I wanted to see a female doctor. So I haven't actually changed GPs but I don't see him any more. And I find this female doctor very, very good, but she doesn't understand haemochromatosis either. But at least she says to

me you know 'I really don't understand what', you know, but I find
that easier to take.

In this account, the combination of diagnostic delay with an apparent lack
of regret or concern expressed for Mary's continuing welfare provoked the
criticism.

Let us now consider the case of Ria Jones, 50, a gardener who has now
retired on medical grounds. She provides a further patient account of the
difficulty of establishing a diagnosis for her symptoms.

AB: So what was the initial phase like, you say severe depression, mood
swings, I mean what was that process like, was it sort of inexplicable?

RJ: Totally inexplicable and it was also quite worrying because never
having been ill but knowing that there was something wrong but no
tests finding out what it is. Because the moment you get a label you
can think, fine, I can work with that, you know, you can do things,
you know it's not your fault, you're not a hypochondriac or anything
like that. Because I felt a hypochondriac but I just knew something
was wrong. And then finally before the, just before the liver biopsy, it
was suggested by my doctor, who was very supportive and you know I
had, I couldn't fault her, but she just didn't know she said 'Well let's
put you on HRT.' And I said 'No, that's not the problem, I just know
that's not the problem.' And before then I'd been offered anti-
depressants and I said 'No that's not the problem either.' And it was
actually quite an uphill struggle saying I am ill but without being able
to pinpoint it.

Ria contends that she had to labour hard to get her claims to a medical
disease given credence. Her need for a label to prove that she was not
turning into a hypochondriac added a sense of urgency to her search for
a medically legitimated diagnosis – although she did not know what
this label would be until the diagnosis was made for her by a medical
practitioner.

In the case of haemochromatosis, therefore, it is not uncommon for
individual patients who have not yet been diagnosed with the condition to
present with non-specific symptoms that could be associated either with
serious medical disorders (such as haemochromatosis or leukaemia), or
with psychiatric disorders such as a depressive illness, or with less deter-
minate conditions such as chronic fatigue syndrome. Once diagnosed, they
may be regarded as anomalies who have presented without the 'proper'
symptoms that are more specific and helpful to the diagnostician. Such
'helpful' patients will be the ones recalled readily as 'proper' cases with the
correct, textbook features of disease (cf Atkinson 1997). If patients with
diffuse or anomalous symptoms are not diagnosed until they present with
classic and advanced symptoms, the 'normal' nosography of the condition

is sustained within the clinical domain, which in turn confirms other symptoms and alternative presentations as anomalous.

One patient, with symptoms that fitted even less clearly into the accepted pattern of haemochromatosis, was Sandra Hutton, a 57-year-old cleaner. She reported inexplicably developing claustrophobia that coincided with the onset of her haemochromatosis symptoms.

SH: No I guess if I have anything I do suffer a lot with now which I never did before is, I'm very claustrophobic, I can't go anywhere. You know whether that's all due to this [haemochromatosis] I don't know. But I mean I never used to be like this, but it's the last …

AB: When did it begin?

SH: This started about two years ago, you know, I mean …

AB: What is your earliest recollection of claustrophobia?

SH: It's got to be when I, about two years ago. It was when I went to have my eye done and they couldn't do the operation, I had to go back in a month and be put out because I went for local [anaesthetic] you know. But they couldn't do it because I panicked too much. So I had to go back then in a month and have it done you know be put to sleep. So that's the first time I've noticed anything like that. Whether that was fright I don't know. But I can't go in a lift.

AB: And it suddenly started happening two years ago?

SH: Yeah, about two or three years ago, about two years, or might be three years. But I can't even go in a lift you know, I mean, I'm terrible. My children, mind, they all laugh, but I mean it's something I just can't help, you know. So whether that's anything to do with this I don't know, you know. But like I said, the joints is the most what I'm concerned about like, and my feet.

The patients in this research perceive their clinical and personal encounters with the disease as fraught with ambiguity and uncertainty, punctuating their everyday engagement with the self, haemochromatosis and medical knowledge (cf. Bharadwaj 2002). In the absence of an inclusive nosography of the disease, individuals frequently encounter clinicians acknowledging the lack of definitive information on personal outcome and disease trajectory. It is therefore common for patients to view clinicians as offering speculative explanations that fail to contain and explain their own erratic ebbs and flows of iron overload. The professional construction of the disease process does not capture their personal experience, nor their own construction of its pathogenesis. Equally, they may find a discrepancy between professional accounts and their own understandings of the links between the disease entity, blood test results, and their own symptoms.

The experience of Ashley, a 47-year-old builder, is particularly telling in this respect.

A: I just don't seem to settle into a steady pattern because the doctor said the one day, 'I can't believe you,' he said, 'you've been low for, low, low, low [iron stores in the blood] and all of a sudden you've bloody jumped.' [high saturation of iron in blood]

AB: Oh, right.

A: He doesn't know why either but …

AB: Right.

A: It [stored iron] doesn't seem to build constantly sometimes. You go, you know, every six, eight weeks it's working roughly, I go up the hospital and you'd expect it to build up at a set level, now it should've settled down, this is what Dr Brown was saying, like. But it doesn't, it seems to be a bit low, a bit low, a bit low, oh nothing will come, come back six weeks, four weeks, whatever, and all of a sudden you go back and it's jumped and I've got to have blood, I'll go back a fortnight later, blood out get it down again.

AB: So it's not at all predictable then?

A: It doesn't seem to be at the moment, no.

When asked how the constant tiredness and listlessness was explained to him by the consultant haematologist he saw on his routine clinic visits, Ashley's response was blunt and to the point.

AB: Have you discussed this issue with the Prof, with the doc? [why you feel so tired]

A: Well I mentioned it but he's not, I don't think he's really up to speed on it and like you say it's, it's such a busy clinic and half the time the blood side, go and do the bloods, and he'll shout out 'What you doing here, bugger off, I'll give you a buzz if your tests are high,' like, you know. So you don't really get the time to sit with him. I don't know whether he'd have the answers anyway. I don't think there's anything he can do about it because if you have any tonics and pick-me-ups they've all got bloomin' iron in, haven't they, most of them.

Richard, 54, an electrical engineer, was similarly caught up in the descriptive uncertainty surrounding his condition.

AB: And did you ask why there's this fluctuation in your ferritin levels, you're saying that it tends to go down to 300 and shoot back up?

R: I asked the, I asked the nurse, she was, she couldn't explain it, who was taking the blood, and I asked … the doctor … and he said he didn't know why but he felt that may be with the levels being so high that the, analytical, there may be some analytical inaccuracies that caused the problem, but felt that once they went down to more reasonable levels that they would stabilise. Now I don't know whether that's true or not, that's all I got.

Classification and experience: expertise, lay beliefs and the doubled discourse

Medical systems across cultures situate control over disease definition, classification, subsequent arrangement and eventual management or treatment in the domain of expertise located either in specific forms of knowledge, institutions, or individuals. In the case of biomedicine, both clinical judgement and laboratory validations of such knowledge claims have become the domain of expertise (Keating and Cambrosio 1994, 2003). Clinical classifications embody expertise in contrast to lay knowledge, and they 'reinforce the separation of the patient from ownership of their condition' (Bowker and Star 1999: 84). Thus it is not uncommon for 'lay' embodied cognition of a disease to remain unacknowledged in the clinical domain, especially in relation to accepted 'expert' laboratory and clinical prognostications.

Bowker and Star (1999) argue that a disease entity is always formally classified in terms of the work that has been done in the laboratory. Clinicians enter the picture at the moment of classification, while the patient rarely does. The determination of a condition that relies on the voice of the patient is marked as a 'suspicious designation'. Thus Bowker and Star conclude that laboratory and clinical perspectives define the real context of disease classification and reinforce the removal of the patient's ownership of their condition (Bowker and Star 1999: 83–4). An illustration of this from our own research is the experience of Richard.

R: I was going away overseas and I said, 'Look, you know if you don't do it now then it's not going to start for months.' And I said, 'Well if you know I've got high iron.' They wanted to do some further tests to prove whether it was genetic or something, and I said, 'Well, if I've got high iron what does it mean, I've got high iron, whether it's genetic or not doesn't really matter, the fact is I've got high iron and we should try and get it down, the reason for it is secondary as far as I'm concerned. Why can't I start venesection now?' And they said, 'Oh there's no rush, there's no hurry, it's not a thing that's just going to, it's not going to make any difference whatsoever.' Alright, it probably wouldn't, but to me I thought, well, I've got a problem, let's get on and sort it out, you know, why do we need to wait for this test which is as far as I could see was fairly academic, and so I tried, actively, I even offered to pay to go private to have it, to start and … a very simple matter to continue. You know they kept saying, 'No, no, no, you wait. … Wait until you see the, go to see the … you know go to the clinic,' and so I literally waited for about months until it got going where I [inaudible] been undergoing this venesection business and getting, and possibly have this, the iron levels sort of brought down. Because I was saying, 'Look, my hands are getting worse literally by the month, by the week, and you're telling me not to do anything and I'm just sort of sitting here. So that was, since then, now that they're doing venesection I can see that something is happening and I'm sort of, I suppose, as content as I could be. Alright, this biopsy thing, I'm on the waiting list, I don't know what that means, I don't know whether that's going to be two weeks, two months, two years, to be honest.'

Richard has not only lost control over the ownership of his condition but his everyday experience of debilitating iron overload is rendered inconsequential by the clinic in need of a laboratory confirmation of the genetic basis to his haemochromatosis.

Scientific nosographic discourses can be contested, however, especially by those who either embody disease or live in close proximity to it. In the case of Down's syndrome, Rayna Rapp (2000) argues for a strong presence of 'doubled discourses' in which scientific (clinical) discourses are contested from various domains of popular knowledge and dispersed into the lives of people directly affected. The notion of clinical discourse, however, is complex. Chatterji *et al.* (1998) argue how, in making up the object called 'clinical discourse', Foucault separated out those who have the right to speak and the institutional sites from which they speak. Thus, according to Chatterji *et al.*, what was not included in this classification of discourses is the speech that breaks through in these very institutional sites despite the agents not having the authority to speak. The authors instead suggest not only that the clinical discourse excludes the subjugated knowledge of the traditional healers or midwives, who are disempowered by the new regime, but that it also excludes the speech of those who come to have a stake in the institutional sites of biomedicine, and that their experience of the clinic is not encoded in the theory of the clinic since it cannot be configured under the notion of resistance (Chatterji *et al.* 1998: 190). Thus individuals like Ria and Richard become important actors from whom a critique of the clinic is performed not so much in the mode of resisting clinical interventions but rather in criticising its obvious inadequacies. These individuals come to exemplify those increasingly numerous voices that break through both within and outside clinical spaces without having the authority to do so. This doubling of discourse is important because it challenges certain taken-for-granted assumptions about the centrality of medicalisation, objectification and dehumanisation to the patients in clinical spaces. What is at stake in this process of contesting clinical classifications from a deeply individuated, self-reflexive and embodied experience of haemochromatosis is the weight and dignity to be assigned to the experiences of the suffering patient by the medical practitioners and their practices in the clinic. The voiced experiences of these patients contest the clinical exclusion of symptoms and signs of disease whose relevance is rejected, or at least questioned, by existing clinical classifications and knowledge systems. Where current clinical knowledge fails to validate the experiences of individual patients, they may either view themselves as hypochondriacs or set about a search for diagnostic labels that can function to normalise the symptoms and naturalise their condition as clinically corroborated. Our research on haemochromatosis shows that this is by no means confined to more overtly contested disease entities such as Chronic Fatigue Syndrome or Gulf War Syndrome.

Conclusion

In her celebrated Manifesto of the Cyborg, Donna Haraway (1990) draws attention to what she calls informatics of domination and the related move from biology as clinical practice to biology as inscription. Communication technologies and biotechnology are crucial tools, she says, which are recrafting our bodies. She implies that medical knowledge has completed an epistemological cycle, from what Foucault (1997) identified as the *Birth of the Clinic* to its eclipse. She argues:

> It is time to write the *Death of the Clinic*. The clinical methods require bodies and work; we have texts and surfaces. Our domina-tions don't work by medicalization and normalization anymore, they work by networking, communications, redesign, stress management. Normalization gives way to automation, utter redundancy.
>
> (Haraway, 1990: 194)

The empirical evidence we have presented renders problematic such claims for a total transformation – from the 'birth' to the 'death' of the clinic. We agree with Chatterji *et al.* (1998) who argue that 'Haraway ignores the very process through which the clinic is maintained both as an idea and a practice in day-to-day functioning in different societal contexts' (Chatterji *et al.* 1998: 171). In the context of haemochromatosis 'the clinic' is far from being rendered redundant by genetic technologies. As we have shown, moreover, patients have a vested interest in affirming the disciplinary modalities of the clinic. They actively seek out 'medicalisation' and 'nor-malisation'. In the process, patients themselves affirm the clinic as the pri-mary site for the legitimation of knowledge and experiences of their condition.

Patients, who feel resentment at the sceptical reception given their claims by professionals, are unable to base their further argument on popular knowledge – as there is none available, given the relative dearth of infor-mation available on the disease – so they then draw on their embodied and multiple experiences of the disease. As they survey their body's everyday response to iron overload and they contest existing clinical assessments, they forge an ambivalent relationship with clinical knowledge. This ongo-ing struggle with the developing clinical understanding of haemochromatosis illustrates how diverse constituencies, such as patients and clinicians, come to have a common vested interest in the disciplines of the clinic. That is to say, haemochromatosis patients come to have a stake in the clinic because it has the authority to objectify and legitimate their condition. Their resistance to the clinic is a desire to be incorporated by the clinic rather than rejected. It does not lead to a simple resistance directed against the medical gaze. More significantly, it is a critique directed at the perceived failure of that gaze to perform its work. This recalls the analysis by Cussins of *ontological choreography*, in which she suggests that a process of objectification in the clinic involves a patient's active participation and self-management as much as management by practitioners (Cussins 1996). In actively pursuing objectification, medicalisation and normalisation, therefore, the individuals in this study are crafting a phenomenology that is not opposed to the emerging definition of the natural history of haemochromatosis: they are actively seeking to contribute to its production. In seeking clinical validation of their experiences of iron overload these individuals demand the active medicalisation and normalisation of their bodies that the clinic has fundamentally failed to achieve in time for them.

It would, therefore, be wrong to assume that patients actively or implicitly resist the medicalisation or the geneticisation of their conditions. As we have seen, the informants we have interviewed have sought actively to engage with the medical definitions of their ill health. It is clear that the haemochromatosis patients we have worked with, notwithstanding their sometimes unsatisfactory experiences of diagnosis, endorse the medical models of their condition. They do not, however, adopt a passive orientation: they seek actively to engage with clinical medicine in order to redefine the boundaries of 'normal' haemochromatosis so as to accommodate their own nosography.

It is, therefore, premature – at best – to assume that new genetic technologies are necessarily and irreversibly transforming the nature of contemporary medicine. There is no doubt that there are processes that lead towards the 'geneticisation' of some conditions, and the identification of genetic risks and susceptibilities is an important ingredient in the identification of some major conditions. But the patients we have interviewed in this study do not experience their inherited haematological problems in this way. Their experienced illness remains firmly within the domain of clinical definitions. The uncertain relationship between genotype and phenotype in this condition – and it is by no means unique in this regard – means that 'geneticisation' remains an unlikely outcome for such patients. From the perspective of the patients we interviewed, the specifically *genetic* character of their condition is of relatively minor importance, compared with the need for accurate and timely clinical diagnosis. The widespread geneticisation of this condition – through population screening, for instance – is likely to reinforce such a view. If the mutation is relatively common and homozygous individuals are readily identified in the population at large, but the penetrance of the gene is highly uncertain and the onset of frank illness may be uncommon, then patients' interests remain in good clinical diagnosis, rather than genetic testing.

Acknowledgements

We acknowledge the financial support of the Economic and Social Research Council (grant no. L218252009). This project was part of the ESRC's Innovative Health Technologies Research Programme. We are grateful to Andrew Webster, the Programme Director, for his support and encouragement. The work was conducted under the aegis of the ESRC Centre for Economic and Social Aspects of Genomics (CESAGen), a collaboration between Lancaster and Cardiff Universities. We are grateful to Mark Worwood, and to other clinical colleagues, and patients – who must remain anonymous – for their help in the conduct of our research.

References

Allen, K. and Williamson, R. (1999) 'Should we genetically test everyone for haemochromatosis?', *Journal of Medical Ethics*, 25: 209–14.
—— (2000) 'Screening for hereditary haemochromatosis – should be implemented now', *British Medical Journal*, 320: 183–4.
Arksey, H. (1994) 'Expert and lay participation in the construction of medical knowledge', *Sociology of Health and Illness*, 16 (4): 448–68.
Atkinson, P. A. (1997) *The Clinical Experience: the construction and reconstruction of medical reality*, 2nd edn. Aldershot: Ashgate.
Atkinson, P. A., Parsons, E. and Featherstone, K. (2001) 'Professional constructions of family and kinship in medical genetics', *New Genetics and Society*, 20 (1): 5–24.
Banks, J. and Prior, L. (2001) 'Doing things with illness: the micro politics of the CFS clinic', *Social Science and Medicine*, 52: 11–23.
Bassett, M. L., Doran, T. J., Halliday, J. W., Bashir, H. V. and Powell, L. W. (1982) 'Idiopathic hemochromatosis: demonstration of homozygous-heterozygous mating by HLA typing of families', *Human Genetics*, 60: 352–6.
Beutler, E., Felitti, V. J., Koziol, J. A., Ho, N. J. and Gelbart, T. (2002) 'Penetrance of 845G-A (C282Y) HFE hereditary haemochromatosis mutation in the USA', *The Lancet*, 359: 211–18.
Bharadwaj, A. (2002) 'Uncertain risk: genetic screening for susceptibility to haemochromatosis', *Health, Risk and Society*, 4 (3): 227–40.
Bharadwaj, A., Prior, L., Clarke A. and Worwood, M. (2006) 'The genetic iceberg', in A. J. Webster (ed.), *Innovative Health Technologies: new perspectives, challenge and critique*. Basingstoke: Palgrave Macmillan.
Bothwell, T. H., Cohen, I., Abrahams, O. L. and Perold, S. M., (1959) 'A familial study in idiopathic hemochromatosis', *American Journal of Medicine*, 27: 730–8.
Bothwell, T. H. and MacPhail, A. P. (1998) 'Hereditary haemochromatosis: etiologic, pathologic and clinical aspects', *Seminars in Hematology*, 35: 55–71.
Bowker, G. C. and Star, L. S. (1999) *Sorting Things Out: classification and its consequences*, Cambridge, MA: MIT Press.

Burke, W., Thomson, E. and Khoury, M. J. (1998) 'Hereditary haemochromatosis: gene discovery and its implications for population-based screening', *Journal of the American Medical Association*, 280 (2): 172–8.

Busby, H., Williams, G. and Rogers, A. (1997) 'Bodies of knowledge: lay and bio-medical understandings of musculoskeletal disorders', in M. A. Elston (ed.), *The Sociology of Medical Science and Technology*. Oxford: Blackwell.

Canguilhem, G. (1989) *The Normal and the Pathological*, trans. Carolyn R. Faw-cett, with an introduction by Michel Foucault. New York: Zone Books.

Chatterji, R., Chattoo, S. and Das, V. (1998) 'The death of the clinic? Normality and pathology in recrafting aging bodies', in M. Shildrick and J. Price (eds), *Vital Signs: Feminist Reconfigurations of the Bio/Logical Body*. Edinburgh: Edinburgh University Press.

Clarke, E. A. (1995) 'Population screening for genetic susceptibility to disease', *British Medical Journal*, 311: 35–8.

Cussins, C. (1996) 'Ontological choreography: agency through objectification in infertility clinics', *Social Studies of Science*, 26: 575–610.

Davis, J. G. (1998) 'Population screening for haemochromatosis: the evolving role of genetic analysis', *Annals of Internal Medicine*, 129: 905–8.

Debre, R. Dreyfus, J.-C., Frezal, J., Labie, D., Lamy, M., Maroteaux, P., Schapira, F. and Schapira, G. (1958) 'Genetics of haemochromatosis', *Annals of Human Genetics*, 23: 16–30.

Epstein, S. (1995) 'The construction of lay expertise: AIDS activism and the forging of credibility in the reform of clinical trials', *Science, Technology and Human Values*, 20 (4): 408–37.

Evans, J., Skrzynia, C. and Burke, W. (2001) 'The complexities of predictive genetic testing', *British Medical Journal*, 322: 1052–6.

Feinstein, A. R. (1967) *Clinical Judgement*. Huntingdon: Krieger.

Finkler, K. (2000) *Experiencing the New Genetics: family and kinship on the medical frontier*. Philadelphia, PA: University of Pennsylvania Press.

Foucault, M. (1997) *The Birth of the Clinic*. London: Routledge.

Haraway, D. (1990) 'A manifesto for cyborgs: science, technology, and socialist feminism in the 1980s', in L. J. Nicholson (ed.), *Feminism/Postmodernism*. London: Routledge.

Harper, P. S. and Clarke, A. (1995) 'An ethical debate: testing may be unhelpful', *British Medical Journal*, 310: 857–8.

Hedgecoe, A. (2003) 'Expansion and uncertainty: cystic fibrosis, classification and genetics', *Sociology of Health and Illness*, 25 (1): 50–70.

—— (2004) 'A reply to Ann Kerr', *Sociology of Health and Illness*, 26 (1): 107–9.

Jackson, H. A., Carter, K., Darke, C., Guttridge, M. G., Ravine, D., Hutton, R. D., Napier, J. A. and Worwood, M. (2001) 'HFE Mutation, iron deficiency and overload in 10,500 blood donors', *British Journal of Haematology*, 114: 474–84.

Keating, P. and Cambrosio, A. (1994) 'Ours is an engineering approach: flow cytometry and the constitution of human t-cell subsets', *Journal of the History of Biology*, 27: 449–79.

—— (2003) 'Real compared to what? Diagnosing leukemias and lymphomas', in M. Lock, A. Young and A. Cambrosio (eds), *Living and Working with the New Medical Technologies*. Cambridge: Cambridge University Press.

Kerr, A. (2000) '(Re)Constructing genetic disease: the clinical continuum between cystic fibrosis and male infertility', *Social Studies of Science*, 30 (6): 847–94.

—— (2004) 'Giving up on geneticization: a comment on Hedgecoe's "Expansion and uncertainty: cystic fibrosis, classification and genetics"', *Sociology of Health and Illness*, 26 (1): 102–6.

Kirmayer, L. J. (1988) 'Mind and body as metaphors: hidden values in biomedicine', in M. Lock and D. R. Gordon (eds), *Biomedicine Examined*. Dordrecht: Kluwer.

McCune, C. A., Al Jader, L. N., May, A., Hayes, S. L., Jackson, H. A. and Worwood, M. (2002) 'Hereditary haemochromatosis: only 1% of adult HFE C282Y homozygotes in South Wales have a clinical diagnosis of iron overload', *Human Genetics*, 111: 538–43.

McDonnell, S. M., Preston, B.L., Jewell, S.A. *et al.* (1999) 'A survey of 2,851 patients with hemochromatosis: symptoms and response to treatment', *American Journal of Medicine*, 106: 619–24

Mishler, E. (1984) *The Discourse of Medicine: dialectics of medical interviews.* Norwood, NJ: Ablex.

Niederau, C., Fischer, R., Purschel, A., Stremmel, W., Haussinger, D. and Strohmeyer, G. (1996) 'Long-term survival in patients with hereditary haemochromatosis', *Gastroenterology*, 110: 1107–19.

Porter, R. (1995) 'The eighteenth century', in L. I. Conrad, M. Neve, V. Nutton, R. Porter and A. Wear (eds), *The Western Medical Tradition 800BC to AD1800.* Cambridge: Cambridge University Press.

Prior, L. (2003) 'Belief, knowledge and expertise: the emergence of the lay expert in medical sociology', *Sociology of Health and Illness*, Silver Anniversary special issue: 41–57.

Rapp, R. (2000) 'Extra chromosomes and blue tulips: Medico-familial interpretations', in M. Lock, A. Young and A. Cambrosio (eds), *Living and Working with the New Medical Technologies.* Cambridge: Cambridge University Press.

Saddi, R. and Feingold, J. (1974) ' Idiopathic haemochromatosis: an autosomal recessive disease', *Clinical Genetics*, 5: 234–41.

Sarangi, S. (2001) 'Demarcating the space between "lay expertise" and "expert laity"' (Editorial), *Text*, 21 (1/2): 3–11.

Seamark, C. J. (2000) 'Should asymptomatic haemochromatosis be treated? Treatment can be onerous for patient and doctor', *British Medical Journal*, 320: 1314–17.

Simon, M., Alexandre, J. L., Bourel, M., Le Marec, B. and Scordia, C. (1977) 'Heredity of idiopathic haemochromatosis: a study of 106 families', *Clinical Genetics*, 11: 327–41.

Waldby, C. (2000) 'Fragmented bodies, incoherent medicine', *Social Studies of Science*, 30 (3): 465–74.

Williamson, R., Allen, K. and Delatycki, M. (2001) 'Haemochromatosis: why we should carry out genetic screening', *World Congress on Iron Metabolism Proceedings*, August 18–23, Cairns, Australia.

Worwood, M. (1999) 'Inborn errors of metabolism: iron', *British Medical Bulletin*, 55: 556–67.

9 Towards an anatomy of public engagement with medical genetics

Robert Evans, Alexandra Plows and Ian Welsh

Introduction

This chapter outlines the anatomy of the emergent – or proto- – politics of genomics, situating primary data gathered within the UK in the context of an increasingly networked social movement milieu (Castells 1996a; Chesters and Welsh 2005; Welsh, *et al.* 2005). In focusing on these nascent moments of social and cultural deliberation we extend the classic conception of politics as the formalisation and expression of interests through representative and administrative institutions to include what Melucci (1989, 1996) has termed 'latency periods'. These periods are the times when emergent'stakes' are actively negotiated as new phenomena begin to challenge existing experiential and analytical categories. Analytically, it is important to recognise that such work typically takes place prior to publicly visible mobilisations as part of a 'shadow realm' (Welsh 2002). In the case of genomic science, the seeds of this political engagement and mobilisation arise from the potential for new techniques and technologies to cut across disciplinary boundaries in both the social and natural sciences, to perturb established conceptual vocabularies and to recast established identities and roles.

EU member states, such as the UK, with a commitment to consultation and transparency, have conducted numerous public engagement exercises amidst increasing attention to the role of health social movements (Brown and Zavestoski 2005). As such, genomics is 'emerging' within a rather different climate to earlier 'big' science advances, such as nuclear power and computing, where major applications were typically formalised before public engagement took place (Radkau 1995; Kepplinger 1995; Nelkin 1995). In contrast, public engagement with genomics is being encouraged and actively sought before major applications are formalised, providing a unique opportunity to 'map' the process of emergence in the context of multi-layered governance approaches.

In approaching these debates, we distinguish between different social actors and institutions (e.g., science, civil society, regulatory agencies) but do not assign any group to one 'side' or another. Instead, we find that members of each group of actors frequently appears in different categories depending on the specific issue or application in question. This in itself is a significant finding, confounding the dualistic pro/anti-positioning that has historically dominated the science and technology literature (Welsh 2000) and suggesting that ambivalence is a defining feature of the process of emergence. We suggest that this process of emergence is marked by significant identity work as the traditional repertoires of political, regulatory and civil society actors encounter unfamiliar challenges. Whilst it may be the case that this ambivalence will become transformed over time into more substantive and simplified forms of political interest representation, this is part of a longer project.

Here, we confine ourselves to presenting the key features of the proto-politics of genomics as issues such as consent, acceptability and scope of application begin to become tangible for individuals and societies (see Habermas 2003). We begin by clarifying how we view the problems of public engagement with what is still a largely unknown quantity. We then provide a tentative social anatomy, in which we distinguish between different types of participants and explore the sometimes unexpected ways in which they find themselves aligning with respect to genomics. Next, we briefly explore the implications of the emerging networks of civil society engagement upon the ways in which genetics can be framed within public debate and conclude by returning to the problem of participation.

Public engagement and the emergence of a proto-politics

Formal politics is associated with rational forms of interest representation, a focus that has been extended to the wider sphere of public administration, with public and planning inquiries assuming increasingly elaborate and extended forms. Wynne (1982) argued that, when faced by complex scientific developments, this focus upon interests is actually irrational because it ignores the question of how individuals can know that they may have an interest in the face of an open-ended techno-scientific development. In Wynne's view the imposition of scientific and judicial forms of substantive rationality effectively co-constructs sharply defined pro and anti positions with active long-term consequences in terms of public acceptability. Initially developed in relation to nuclear power, these arguments have subsequently been highly influential in foregrounding issues of public acceptance and consultation *sui generis*. Indeed, in the genomic sphere, where the societal implications of genetic screening, selection, therapeutic intervention and enhancement are significant and 'timeless', the techno-scientific trajectories remain open-ended and indeterminate. The 'upstream' consequences in terms of technical, social and moral 'risks' intertwine with the quest for public consultation and consensus representing a bulwark against rejection and antipathy.

The focus of these consultations cannot just be about the technical and scientific aspects of genomics, however. Habermas (2003) argues that, without direct attention to explicitly moral categories, the incremental pursuit of genomic techniques will undermine any notion of 'species-being', as human nature becomes a site of scientific intervention alongside nature *qua* the environment. Whilst Habermas broadly accepts the medical and therapeutic potential of genomics, he argues that the potential for genetic enhancement, screening and parental genetic selection requires wide-ranging public debate prior to their availability. Once such techniques become available they will undermine a universal element of the human condition – the chances of birth – a shared ontological status forming the basis for the exercise of collective moral judgement. Habermas effectively argues that such normative considerations provide a *firmer* basis for the development of genomics than a narrow prioritisation of scientific and technological knowledge, which is ultimately *contingent* in such a rapidly evolving field.

The challenge formalised philosophically here is formidable in terms of established notions of interest representation and the means of incorporating such interests within decisional and policy-making processes. This is implicitly acknowledged in the view that, in order to avoid 'being an *overpowering* consensus', any agreement must 'integrate the entire complexity of the objections *reasonably refuted* as well as the unrestricted variety of interests and interpretive perspectives that *were taken into account*' (Habermas 2003: 57).

For our purposes the importance of these arguments revolves around the notion of 'unrestricted variety of interests and interpretive perspectives'. Such an open-ended commitment inevitably raises questions about the ways in which these voices can be articulated within public debate and consultation. For example, which social actors are carriers of embodied moral knowledge that is relevant for the choices made possible by genomics? How are these voices to be 'weighed' in relation to those of general publics, technical and scientific stakeholders and the operation of market forces? One indication of the difficulty this commitment raises can be seen in the concern with inter-generational equity which inevitably arises as individuals make choices over the genetic configuration of the as yet unborn.

These are, of course, precisely the sorts of questions which have given ethics such a prominent place in the consideration of the new genetics whilst simultaneously exceeding the analytical capacity of liberal formulations grounded in an abstract individual (Glasner and Rothman 2001). Here we outline some expressions of the kinds of ambivalent stances held in a variety of social positions, identifying some initial sites where these questions are starting to be grappled with. This data suggests that the proto-politics of genomics contains high levels of ambiguity for both 'producers' and 'consumers' of genetic knowledge alike, producing unexpected 'issue' alliances or 'strange bed-fellows'.

Social anatomy: producer/entrepreneur/citizen

Genomics constitutes a double challenge in terms of the alignment of scientific practitioners with the process of innovation. First, there is a radical reconfiguration of disciplinary boundaries with implications for professional esteem, grant eligibility and public standing. Second, genomic techniques are firmly located within a neo-liberal framework emphasising the early transfer of viable techniques to the private sector and the alignment of public- and private-sector initiatives through 'collaboratories'. The spread of co-funding, enterprise units and university biotech start-up companies thus compromises the ideotypic view of the university as the natural repository of independent expert advice (Kenney 1986). Entrepreneurial science, associated with the 'third way' in the UK, reconfigures familiar tensions between state secrecy and scientists' freedom to publish results, with issues of commercial secrecy and competitive advantage becoming increasingly salient.

Such factors impact upon the experience of identity at all levels of the scientific workforce. Interview data show that the ideotypic self-identity of the scientist as a key actor in securing progress and human advancement that was associated with positive recruitment to earlier 'big science' breakthroughs (Welsh 2000) is attenuated within the genomic workforce. Once-positive images are now being replaced by ambiguity, and these tensions are amplified by the dominance of computer-mediated communication and the interdisciplinary interpretation, formalisation and application of knowledge, all of which are key factors in the process of innovation. A key tension embedded within this formalisation lies in the distinction between information and knowledge (Lash 2002; Chesters and Welsh 2006). In this emergent milieu, the apparent solidity and security of clearly demarcated disciplinary and social identities is perturbed by entry into liquid modernity, life in fragments and the fluid self (Bauman 2000, 1995). The contemporary emphasis on governance and consultation takes place as citizenhood and citizenship are increasingly experienced and acted upon in terms of multiple selves prioritised through context and situated relevance (Turner 2001). In terms of an emergent proto-politics of genomics, the resultant 'strange bed-fellows' identified here reflect *both* the technical and the social assemblages which increasingly shape public–science relations (Irwin and Michael 2003).

In terms of scientists' selves, these tensions are reflected in our data in relation to a wide range of substantive areas, including the transition from 'wet bench work' to 'dry mathematical modelling', pressures for open-access data exchange and associated issues relating to patenting. The following cases highlight some of the more important areas where tensions in the scientist–citizen–innovation process co-construct ambivalence and bring about some counterintuitive issue alliances.

From wet to dry: evaporating disciplines, crystallising new networks

One way in which the development of genomic science challenges established boundaries between categories of scientific work can be seen in the nature of biological research. Here, the traditional view of biology as a 'wet' science based on laboratory bench work using chemical and other assays is melded with an emphasis on the use of computer models and other mathematical approaches. This paradigm shift changes both the nature of research work in those biological sciences associated with genomics, which 'become a "theoretical" science' (Hilgartner 1995: 302), and the relationship between biology and other disciplines.

In some ways, the move to more mathematical, computational modelling approaches can be seen to diminish the prestige of the work by constituting the subject as a service provided to others rather than an innovative field in its own right. In this sense some of the most important 'science wars' take place between natural science disciplines. Thus, for example, some of our respondents predicted the disappearance of some areas of research within the bio-sciences:

> it depends on whether you see bionomics as a discipline in itself or just as a tool box ... some people are saying bionomics is a discipline and predicting that it will get bigger whereas other people are predicting [it] will disappear. As standard computers have got faster then biology isn't the same.
>
> (Gene sequencer, Sanger Institute)

Others see the shift to more mathematical and computational kinds of bioscience as a major opportunity. As biotechnology becomes based in the practices of computing and mathematical modelling, the move away from established disciplinary practices is accompanied by a move into other scientific domains, particularly those of nanotechnology and information technology. The consequences of this gradual blurring and merging of traditionally separate disciplines raises potential problems as it becomes increasingly difficult to categorise and thus to regulate genomic innovations:

> If you go ten, fifteen years into the future, you're not going to be able to distinguish between what's nanotechnology, what's biotechnology and what's genetic engineering ... and there is a lot of politics of control, who controls it ... who's being excluded.
>
> ('Mike', GM activist/ETC group)

In terms of Habermas's prescription to articulate all relevant perspectives, the fluidity of genomic science thus raises significant challenges, as establishing clear technical boundaries between both knowledge domains and potential applications becomes increasingly difficult. As a result, the 'single "postbox"' (Jasanoff 1995: 321) style of regulation favoured within the UK is likely to struggle in the face of the cross-cutting nature of genomics.

The problem of categorisation is not the only one faced by regulatory agencies, however. As noted above, genomic research often takes place in a quasi-commercialised environment, and our data suggest that the predominance of market values adds a further significant dimension to issues of trust.

> [T]here's like professors in labs, like in nine times out of ten if you're the head of a lab that's working on a human disease it's a culture of entrepreneurialism. You're going to have these conflicts of interest. And they are going to introduce bias, you know, whether it's unconscious or whatever, it's just not right to have those associations.
>
> (Mike, GM activist/ETC Group)

In this instance the experience of the corporate deployment of science within GM could be a significant frame for both regulators and critics. Interestingly, however, our data also reveal similar concerns amongst the professional associations representing scientific workers, suggesting that this is a much broader concern (Welsh *et al.* 2005).

Prominent examples of concern over market values within the scientific workforce can be seen in the preference of some researchers to approach genomic data as 'open-source'. Mathematical expressions of genomic knowledge facilitate electronic dissemination and raise significant issues for the ownership and control of innovation. Once mounted in an open-access domain, multiple agents can reconfigure, refine and augment the original work, producing new and unanticipated outputs. The potential benefits for citizens of such 'open-source' genomic knowledge are balanced against both commercial and professional arguments for proprietorial approaches towards knowledge. One such 'citizen scientist' provides a particularly clear formalisation.

> I find that ... the division between protestors and activists and academics is really artificial and a lot of the people I met [at the Sanger institute] are like activists; ... I started to talk about [the] politics of open access and stuff like that [and] people are completely clued up ... Those same people could walk into jobs paying like fifty, sixty, seventy grand a year. They're not; they're conscientiously going into this open source movement ... what I like to do now is a matter of just putting the data out and putting tools at people's disposal.
>
> ('Alice', genetic sequencer, Sanger Institute, November 2003)

In summary, therefore, the emerging bio-science field, with its developing emphasis on computational approaches, has the potential to challenge the traditional categories of scientific, commercial and regulatory institutions.

As such, any proto-politics of genomic research will find itself ranging over a heterogeneous set of issues, concerns and institutions and, as we explore in more detail in the following sections, this can give rise to some unexpected alliances.

Patenting life or securing progress: corporates for open access?

The cross-cutting nature of genomic science and the potential to generate strange alliances features prominently in the area of patenting. It might be expected that scientific and commercial interests would broadly support patenting as means of consolidating research findings and securing a return on investment. As we show below, although this is just how patenting is often presented, there are also exceptions.

At the launch of the Danish Council of Ethics (2004) report *Patenting Human Genes and Stem Cells*, the opening address by the Rector of the University of Copenhagen, Linda Nielsen, presented patenting as an established, tried and tested means of ensuring that the benefits of progress became widely available through the commercial application of scientific and technical advances. Without such commercial reward the ensuing medical benefits associated with biotechnology would not become available. Patenting was an area where the public required 'expert guidance', as it lay outside commonsense understanding and could only be clarified and resolved through the engagement of 'independent experts'. The address thus sought to foreclose the notion of biotechnological advance being predicated on the patenting of 'life' in the abstract – a move inimical to the open engagement envisaged by Habermas.

In contrast, out data suggest that this traditional approach to patenting will be challenged by a variety of social groups and stakeholders questioning the distinction between 'ownership' as an absolute category and the temporally limited 'control' of biological material. Our data reveal that patenting is an area where there is no simple, expert consensus about its utility or acceptability, and that this ambivalence extends into both the commercial and the scientific domains, as the following quotes illustrate.

> There should be no patenting of gene sequences, period. They were invented by nature.
>
> (Affymetrix, US biotech company, March 2003)

> The intellectual property arena is nothing less than a minefield. If a genesequence is patented, you can't necessarily design around it. What type of discovery associated with the gene sequence would entitle somebody to lock up a whole area of research and prevent competition?
>
> (Dr Elliot Sigal, Senior Vice President of Early Discovery and Applied Technology, Bristol-Myers Squibb's Pharmaceutical Research Institute.)

Whilst expressions of concern such as these from within commercial and scientific sites could be interpreted in terms of commercial/self-interest, they also reflect the cross-cutting nature of genomic research. The widely anticipated arrival of clear-cut genetic therapies has yet to be realised. Instead, genomics has revealed very few single gene conditions and a multitude of complex co-causative chains. Granting exclusive patent rights to one particular application thus risks foreclosing other equally important applications. In this sense the problematic identity of genomic science as certainty is rendered complex and indeterminate (Wynne 2005). Despite this, 4,382 human genes, almost 20 per cent of the human genome, are the subject of US patents, with some genes being the subject of up to twenty patent applications (Jensen and Murray 2005). Almost half of these patents reside with a single company, Incyte Pharmaceuticals/Incyte Genomics.

Within Europe a number of alternatives to patenting have been advanced as a means of overcoming some of these issues. These include the application of a 'copy-right' or licensing approach enabling multiple applications subject to a fee. In the case of stem cell lines for therapeutic interventions, registration of significant patient groups as co-patent holders in applications targeting their particular condition has also been proposed. Significantly, these debates divide a variety of 'expert' communities and open up multiple lines of affiliation that, in turn, resonate with a variety of civil society actors. As a result, a diverse range of civil society, scientific and regulatory actors are engaging with these issues and producing multiple interest representations (see EGE 2000, 2002). Before illustrating key frames generated by these actors, it is important to emphasise that the implications of the prevailing neo-liberal axiomatic represent a significant theme in the responses of scientists and practitioners at a variety of levels. These range from statements at a high level of abstraction such as:

> I think that – a lot of the body of the risk associated with genetic technology actually comes from the capitalist structure underlying the usage of that technology ... if you were to offer that technology in a democratic way then all the issues about ... insurance and haves and have nots, would go away. If everybody was entitled to the best, then those issues wouldn't exist.

... to recognition of the impact of 'third way' flexible labour market strategies on the scientific work force. Here, gendered identity is a particularly significant feature, with some young women abandoning their science careers to enter occupations in which contractual relations are compatible with parenthood (see Welsh *et al.* 2005, Welsh 2006).

Civil society: the importance of social movements

As part of the wider biotechnology sector, human genomic techniques (i.e. red genomics) are conventionally located within an assemblage of applications, including GM crops (green genomics), with plant species being used as hosts for genetic material from a range of animal sources. The way in which the genomic assemblage spans the plant–animal divide could be problematic given the difficulties experienced by proponents of agricultural biotechnology in the EU. As Salter and Jones (2002: 337) observe:

> Although the body politic of human genetics and health may at present appear to be unaffected by the political virus which has so virulently attacked green biotechnology, it would be unwise to assume immunity.

The same authors underline the reported difficulty of finding respondents to public consultation initiatives. Despite this apparent lack, we were able to identify a range of civil society actors, ranging from 'the usual suspects' like Greenpeace and Genewatch to dedicated citizens' groups and a growing number of patients' groups. The prevailing social movement milieu is thus composed of groups which might be reasonably expected to have an established 'path-dependent' orientation towards red genetics and a range of emergent groups engaged in the process of sense-making associated with emergence and latency periods. This process of framing and the declaration of 'collective stakes' (Melucci 1996) takes place within an era in which participation in social movement actions and the adoption of social movement repertoires of action by increasingly diverse social groups has been interpreted as heralding the rise of the social movement society (Meyer and Tarrow 1998). For present purposes, what is important is the situated framing by a diversity of actors as envisaged by Habermas, and the acknowledgement and accommodation of the complexity of views expressed irrespective of their acceptance or refutation.

A science that explicitly promises to cure genetic disorders also poses a threat to those with identities founded upon their particular allocation of genetic life chances. Our data contain numerous examples of the resultant ambivalence and prioritisation of forms of choice which are difficult to incorporate within existing ethical frameworks. The following selections illustrate key stances represented within the data set.

> We had a pre-existing group which formed on crops and genetics and when we heard about the Centre for Life coming to Newcastle, we thought we had to do something. But we didn't have much of a plan, so we ended up mostly reacting to their publicity days ... At the time we weren't very sure what it [the Centre for Life] was. It was billed as being a massive kind of investment showcase for genetics ... there was very little of it rented already, so we were guessing whether it was going to be animal labs or whether it was going to be offices even, for non-associated companies ... We weren't quite sure which

ethical issues were going to be in the forefront, so we spent quite a lot of time just casting about for ideas really for what to do. We felt it was our responsibility to do something, but it wasn't our main concern at the time.

(Interview with M1)

[On disability groups] affected by eugenics ... they're dealing with their own death. They're basically seen as defective and abnormal and that, having the technology in place to eradicate them ... they may become no longer wanted.

('Mike', GM activist/ETC group)

Given the small number of single gene disorders that have been discovered and for which tests are available, such ambivalence intensifies when confronted by genetic diagnostics expressed in terms of 'a propensity' towards a particular condition. Such unease is perhaps compounded by the clinical advice for radical mastectomy which has tended to accompany diagnosis of a genetic propensity for breast cancer. Irrespective of this possible association, any move to establish abortion as a normative response in the face of a potential genetic condition will be contested in terms of a right to difference. This is a form of choice which does not fit easily with universal liberal rights such as those espoused within the UK's HGC.

We affirm that humans are born equal, that they are entitled to equality of opportunity, and that neither genetic constitution nor genetic knowledge should be used to limit that equality [which] should be incorporated into UK legislation and practice.

(Sir John Sulston, HGC, *The Guardian* 15.05.04: 1)

Such stances are also difficult to reconcile with the view of scientific progress and medical cure, not to mention neo-liberal market logic. The counterpoint is that humans are born *different* and, as sentient, conscious human beings, have an equal right to exercise choice.

Genomics, identity and governance

These ethical dilemmas arising from the claims made for genomic science raise difficult questions for regulators and wider society, precisely because of the ambivalence they engender and the uncertain consequences associated with such innovations over time. Whilst scientific practitioners tend to emphasise the importance of medical and therapeutic techniques enabled by this science, longer-term issues include genetic enhancement and the social desirability of substantially extending human life. The analytical distinction between therapeutic applications and enhancement is problematic given the potential for multiple applications arising from common techniques. To date, ethical considerations have tended to focus on front-end issues relating to access to human biological materials (Welsh 2006). As a result, the wide-ranging debate about 'up-stream' stakes identified as crucial by Habermas remains noticeable by its absence.

In terms of promissory identities associated with genomics, these are issues already established within the public sphere. The respected BBC2 documentary series *Horizon*, for example, included medical scientists' claims that 'death can now be regarded as an illness' which in the future 'may be cured' ('Life & Death in the 21st Century', Part 1, 4 January 2000). Genetic enhancement is a topic included in public consultation exercises and reported in relation to the future of athletic competition (e.g. BBC1's Ten O'Clock News, 17 February 2004).

Like promissory statements made in relation to previous scientific breakthroughs, such claims can assume considerable significance when they are 'time-shifted' (Welsh 2000). Given the increasing ease with which such time-shifting can be accomplished in a digital age, yesterday's 'heroic' scientific announcement can become tomorrow's Achilles heel. Salter and Jones conclude that the legitimacy of 'red' biotechnology would struggle to 'survive prolonged public exposure to a media-driven issue in human genetics' (Salter and Jones 2002: 338).

The vulnerability of genomics to contamination by association with GM and a human application controversy haunts regulatory and consultative initiatives. In terms of identity and the data presented here, some clear themes emerge. In particular, whilst Habermas's notion of full consultation cannot guarantee enhanced public acceptance for genomic science, it offers a basis for a robust defence of the legitimacy of decisions taken at a particular time. Tolerance of diverse identities linked to meaningful up-stream influence within a range of consultative and regulatory fora thus assume a position of some importance.

Public engagement with/through/by civil society

There is increasing recognition of the capacity for organised citizen groups to make substantive contributions to regulatory science and regulatory standards (Epstein 1996, Tesh 2000). In part these refinements to scientific knowledge arise from the adoption of citizen standpoints which configure stakes through 'logics' different to those of bench or theoretical scientists. They are also part of the process of negotiated moral standards applied to science as an expression of material culture (Jasper 1997), and it is in this wider sense that Habermas's call for recognition of complexity should be read. In the case of genomics, a diversity of knowledges and moral frames constitutes the flows configuring the 'emergence of particular blocs' that 'cut across scientific, commercial, civic, regulatory, media and lay sectors' constituting what Irwin and Michael term 'ethno-epistemic assemblages' (Irwin and Michael 2003: 112–13).

Genomics thus poses significant challenges for both the natural and the social sciences. These can be seen most clearly in responses to the UK's *GM Nation?* debate, which raised issues of sampling public responses (Horlick-Jones *et al.* 2004). Expressed concisely, these revolve around the difference in responses between those termed the 'active participants' and a randomised set of respondents, referred to as the 'Narrow but Deep' sample and chosen to represent the 'silent majority'. Significantly the evaluation of questions relating to issues such as 'future benefits' was central to this debate and, in these issues, the 'self-selecting' active participants in the *GM Nation?* sample exhibited greater scepticism than the 'random' sample. The critique of the *GM Nation?* sample overlooks not only the long-established point that greater public knowledge can increase scepticism but also the cross-cutting nature of genomic techno-science which inevitably co-constructs multiple public–citizen science–scientific citizen standpoints.

Periods of proto-political emergence are marked by the existence of multiple counterintuitive alignments between strange bed-fellows operating within increasingly open networked systems. The critical question for social science embedded within this process of emergence is whether it is more important to identify and listen to the voices of what may be termed 'critical sub-groups' (i.e. the 'active participants') or to assess the stance of general publics (i.e. the 'Narrow but Deep' sample). Habermas is implicitly suggesting that the general democratic will of the body politic can only engage with genomics by taking critical sub-groups seriously. There is much to commend this view if the alternative is an incremental journey towards the 'neo-liberal eugenics' he fears.

For representative democracy the distinction between government and governance (multi-layered or otherwise) remains opaque in terms of the impact of governance initiatives, including public consultation exercises, upon the outputs of government. Governance initiatives, like *GM Nation?*, operate as point attracters producing patterned, self-selecting participants. Processes of emergence are strongly associated with the operation of strange attracters (Chesters and Welsh 2005) and the strange bed-fellow clusters identified here can be thought of as expressions of this process.

The reduction of this complexity to pro–anti/for-us-or-against-us binaries through the imposition of established categories and concepts, including economic interest, appears to politically pre-judge issues before the generation, formalisation and expression of the socially complex 'grounds for concern' over genomic science reaches an equilibrium position. For Habermas, such an equilibrium position might be reached through a considered process of carefully weighed statements by diverse protagonists. In terms of social interaction this translates as listening carefully to individuals with *queer* identities speaking in unfamiliar tongues as part of the engagement with risk *and* identity (McKechnie and Welsh 2002).

A range of commentators have criticised social movement theorists for paying insufficient attention to the primary framing of grassroots activists and prioritising that of movement intellectuals (Tesh 2000). Such cases are particularly important when there is a transition from community concern and action towards a social movement orientation (Bauman 2001; Lichterman 1996). Gaining access to such primary framing during periods of emergence is particularly critical, as these are moments when the work of latency periods begins to be expressed. Such expressions regularly take unfamiliar forms readily marginalised as 'deviant' or 'anti-science' (Chesters and Welsh 2006). This makes the creation and maintenance of open social boundary conditions for public consultation processes a critical factor. Exclusion and 'empty' incorporation increase the social distance between publics and science. Academic work has shown that the new genetics is an area where focus group participants demonstrate a sophisticated appreciation of the stakes and recognise the need to draw certain lines (Kerr *et al.* 1998). Given the capacity of publics to draw such lines within the sheltered confines of focus groups, a critical question becomes, how are such boundaries drawn in terms of lived relations and situated practices?

Conclusions

In this chapter we have examined the proto-politics of genomics developing outside the formal institutions of representative democracy and governance initiatives. In doing so, we have implicitly recognised the capacity of civil society actors to challenge dominant discourses and reframe the ways in which science, technology and indeed politics are being recast in the context of increasingly global flows. In this way, we are following Touraine (1981) and Melucci (1989, 1996) in emphasising the importance of the symbolic dimension of scientific and technological innovation. It is not just what genomics can do in the laboratory that matters, but the implications of using these techniques outside the laboratory for the distribution of power, inclusion, equity and justice within society. These concerns assume a new significance, as Touraine's (1983) insight that science is no longer dependent upon the state is accentuated within an ascendant neo-liberal globalisation.

The problem for civil society actors, organisations and wider lay publics is that making sense of a new cross-cutting science such as genomics, with implications for both new medical procedures and human species being, is no easy task. For scientists and regulators and many engaged citizens it is a full-time job. It is for this reason that we began by emphasising the importance of the 'latency periods' identified by Melucci in which formalised and emergent movement actors work to identify *both* specific *and* collective stakes.

This hidden work is crucial because it represents a frequently overlooked phase of engagement in which the debate is typically far more wide-ranging and proactive than studies of formalised pro- and anti-controversies suggest. Social movements thus aim to selectively modernise rather than reject modern values (Offe 1985). Confronted by such challenges, established political and administrative institutions effectively reduce complexity through the imposition of familiar categories *producing* pro–anti binaries. In this way the social innovation of critical sub-groups, broadly understood as social movements, is set in opposition to the transformatory potential of science rather than being included in the co-construction of progress.

The proto-politics of genomic science occurs within increasingly global networks as the global regulatory reach (Welsh and Evans 1999; Welsh 2000) associated with techno-science and neo-liberal economics has become increasingly prominent. Whilst formal genomic consultation initiatives have had difficulty in finding participants, we have demonstrated the existence of a wide range of formalised, informal and network actors actively engaged in sense-making around the new genetics. This is consistent with Touraine's invocation that social movement research should be conducted as close as possible to sites of activity, paying attention to both the formalisation of specific grievances and the wider associated stakes (Touraine 1981).

The critical claim that we make in this chapter is that the process of emergence, through which public stakes and issues are developed, is an important part of civil society engagement with genomics. To focus upon formally constituted participants is to miss an important dimension of the problem. In particular, to the extent that established 'core antagonistic actors' define the issues and stakes, then they act to close rather than to open up debate by working within the established frames set by representative democratic institutions. Here, the dominant primary frame has become technical risk (Beck 1992) which has tended to elevate knowledge claims to a position of prominence, leading Bauman to regard this as 'technocracy's last stand' (Bauman 1993: 207).

Our data suggest that the neo-liberal context within which genomic science is being introduced represents an area of significant concern on both sides of the producer/consumer divide. This is redolent of Castells's argument that neo-liberalism is the over-arching concern forming the basis for global collective solidarity expressed through multiple social movements (Castells 1996b). Combined with notions of iteration, central to complexity theory, there is thus a potential for paradigmatic change distinct from cycles-of-contention approaches. The presence of counterintuitive alliances composed of strange bed-fellows is historically associated with such phase shifts in social systems (Chesters and Welsh 2006). Our distinction between established and emergent movement actors provides not only a more accurate description of what is happening but directs attention towards some significant nodes within the emergent nested networks.

An adequate public engagement with genomics, if it is to happen, must seek to involve a wide range of actors, including some *queer* folk, if it is to articulate the range of views, stakes and meanings attributed to genomics within society. Including a wide range of movements and organisations would widen the range of discourses used to debate genomics. Dominant rhetorics of progress, cure and choice would be complemented and/or contested by those of social justice, commodification and discrimination that declare the collective moral and ethical stakes embedded within the conventional technical frame. These are stakes clearly articulated around patenting where balancing individual and collective benefits assumes a key position. In terms of our data, concerns around business ethics, the sanctity and integrity of the body, and scientific freedom to innovate are significant themes.

In emphasising these aspects of a techno-scientific innovation, emergent social movements thus highlight the symbolic and cultural stakes associated with the application of genetics in different fields. In doing so they challenge the taken-for-granted frameworks of scientific and regulatory institutions and, potentially, perturb the networks of support they draw on. They also act as a catalyst for wider deliberation and change consistent with notions of deliberative democracy (Dryzek 2000). Bringing these ideas and perspectives to the fore within critical civil society has the potential to promote public and regulatory engagement with genomics that recognises it as a source of social innovation and not just an application of techno-scientific progress.

Finally, it is important to be clear what follows from this new description. First, it does not adopt a position that is either for or against genomics. Rather, we are suggesting that what is needed is a way of thinking about and managing the relationships between science and society that enables civic deliberation to take place. In particular, it suggests that there are two important symmetries that need to be recognised if the kind of inclusive deliberation that includes the 'unrestricted variety of interests and interpretive perspectives' highlighted by Habermas is to take place.

The first symmetry is that technical knowledge is not the exclusive preserve of the scientific community. Scientists clearly do have access to specialist knowledge and experience that is not widely shared, but this is also true of other groups. This is particularly obvious in the case of genetic screening, but the point is far more general. In particular, focusing on experience and engagement as the basis for knowledge permits a far more inclusive approach, even to the scrutiny of technical knowledge. In this sense there are within wider communities individuals and organisations who are knowledgeable experts in their own right (Evans and Plows 2005).

The second symmetry runs the other way, and emphasises the ways in which science itself is a kind of social movement with a distinctive set of values and goals (Yearley 1988). Science in this sense is never reducible to whatever the state or big business wants it to be. Rather, science pursues knowledge and technological innovations that aim to make a difference in the world, differences which have moral and ethical aspects as well as technical ones. Debating the moral worthiness and ethical justice associated with such advances, and in particular the desirability of particular classes of applications, may well become increasingly important as the claims made for genomics yield applications requiring regulation. Given the ambivalence that many of these applications currently engender and the impossibility of putting the genie back into the bottle, there is a compelling case for arguing, as Habermas does, that explicit and serious consideration of the moral and ethical stances associated with genomics is an urgent requirement. Within this the universal presence of human difference (rather than liberal notions of equality) represents an axiomatic starting point. Combined with an emphasis upon the situated expressions of affected individuals and groups with direct experience of contested domains, the dialogical negotiation of progress between critical sub-groups, general publics, epistemic communities, and political, economic and regulatory elites becomes a possibility. The exercise of informed choice in these complex areas is necessary to avoid the *de facto* imposition of a market driven or techno-rationalistic 'genetic control or influence over the basic constitution of an individual' (Habermas 1968/1971: 117).

References

Bauman, Z. (1993) *Postmodern Ethics*. Oxford: Blackwell.
—— (1995) *Life in Fragments: essays in post-modern morality*. Oxford: Oxford University Press.
—— (2000) *Liquid Modernity*. Cambridge: Polity.
—— (2001) *Community: seeking safety in an insecure world*. Cambridge: Polity.
Beck, U. (1992) *Risk Society: towards a new modernity*. London: Sage.
Brown, P. and Zavestoski, S. (2005) 'Social movements in health: an introduction', *Sociology of Health & Illness* 26 (6): 679–94.
Castells, M. (1996a) 'The rise of the network society', Volume 1 of *The Information Age: Economy, Society and Culture*. Oxford: Blackwell.
—— (1996b) 'The power of identity', Volume 2 of *The Information Age: economy, society and culture*. Oxford: Blackwell.
Chesters, G. and Welsh, I. (2005) 'Complexity and social movement(s): process and emergence in planetary action systems', *Theory Culture & Society*, 22 (5): 187–211.
—— (2006) *Complexity and Social Movement: multitudes on the edge of chaos*. London: Routledge.
Danish Council of Ethics (2004) *Patenting Human Genes and Stem Cells: a report*. Can be obtained from http://www.etiskraad.dk (accessed 21 July 2006).
Dryzek, J. S. (2000) *Deliberative Democracy and Beyond: liberals, critics and contestations*. Oxford: Oxford University Press.
EGE (2000) *Citizens Rights and New Technology: a European challenge*. Brussels: European Group on Ethics in Science and New Technologies.
—— (2002) *A History of Patenting Life in the United States with Comparative Attention to Europe and America*. Brussels: European Group on Ethics in Science and New Technologies.
Epstein, S. (1996) *Impure Science: AIDS activism and the politics of science*. Berkeley, CA: University of California Press.
Evans, R. J., and Plows, A. (forthcoming) 'Listening without prejudice: rediscovering the value of the disinterested citizen', *Social Studies of Science*, accepted August 2006.

Ganchoff, C. (2005). 'Regenerating movement: embryonic stem cells and the politics of potentiality', *Sociology of Health & Illness*, 26 (6): 757–74.

Glasner, P. and Rothman, H. (2001) 'New genetics, new ethics? Globalisation and its discontents', *Health, Risk & Society*, 3 (3): 245–59.

Habermas, J. (1968/1971) *Towards a Rational Society*. London: Heinemann.

—— (2003) *The Future of Human Nature*. Oxford: Polity.

Hilgartner, S. (1995) 'The human genome project', in S. Jasanoff, G. E. Markle, J. C. Petersen and T. Pinch (eds), *Handbook of Science and Technology Studies*. London: Sage.

Horlick-Jones, T., Walls, J., Rowe, G., Pidgeon, N., Poortinga, W. and O'Riordan, T. (2004) *A Deliberative Future? An Independent Evaluation of the GM Nation? Public Debate about the Possible Commercialisation of Transgenic Crops in Britain, 2003*, Understanding Risk Working Paper 04–02, University of East Anglia. Available online at http://www.uea.ac.uk/env/pur/gm_future_top_copy_12_feb_04.pdf (accessed 11 August 2004).

Irwin, A. and Michael, M. (2003) *Science, Social Theory and Public Knowledge*. Maidenhead: Open University Press.

Jasanoff, S. (1995) 'Product, process, or programme: three cultures and the regulation of biotechnology', in M. Bauer (ed.), *Resistance to New Technology: nuclear power, information technology and biotechnology*. Cambridge: Cambridge University Press.

Jasper, J. M. (1997) *The Art of Moral Protest: culture, biography and creativity in social movements*. Chicago, IL: Chicago University Press.

Jensen, K. and Murray, F. (2005) 'Enhanced: intellectual property landscape of the human genome', *Science*, 310 (5746): 239–40.

Kenney, M. (1986) *Biotechnology: the university–industrial complex*. New Haven, CT: Yale University Press.

Kepplinger, H. M. (1995) 'Individual and institutional impacts on press coverage of sciences: the case of nuclear power and genetic engineering in Germany', in M. W. Bauer (ed.), *Resistance to New Technology: nuclear power, information technology and biotechnology*. Cambridge: Cambridge University Press.

Kerr A., Cunningham Burly, S. and Amos, A. (1998) 'Drawing the line: an analysis of lay people's discussions about the new genetics', *Public Understanding of Science*, 7: 113–33.

Lash, S. (2002) *Critique of Information*. London: Sage.

Lichterman, P. (1996) *The Search for Political Community: American activists reinventing commitment*. Cambridge: Cambridge University Press.

McKechnie, R. and Welsh, I. (2002) 'When the global meets the local: critical reflections on reflexive modernisation', in F. Buttel, P. Dickens, R. Dunlap and A. Gijswijt (eds), *Sociological Theory and the Environment: classical foundations, contemporary insights*. Boulder, CO: Rowman & Littlefield.

Melucci, A. (1989) *Nomads of the Present*. London: Radius Hutchinson.

—— (1996) *Challenging Codes: collective action in the information age*. Cambridge: Cambridge University Press.

Meyer, D. S. and Tarrow, S. (eds) (1998) *The Social Movement Society: contentious politics for a new century*. Oxford: Rowman & Littlefield.

Nelkin, D. (1995) 'Forms of intrusion: comparing resistance to information technology and biotechnology in the USA', in M. W. Bauer (ed.), *Resistance to New Technology: nuclear power, information technology and biotechnology*. Cambridge: Cambridge University Press.

Offe, C. (1985) 'New social movements: challenging the boundaries of institutional politics', *Social Research*, 2 (4): 817–68.

Radkau, J. (1995) 'Learning from Chernobyl for the fight against genetics? Stages and stimuli of German protest movements – a comparative synopsis', in M. W. Bauer (ed.), *Resistance to New Technology: nuclear power, information technology and biotechnology*. Cambridge: Cambridge University Press.

Salter, B. and Jones, M. (2002) 'Regulating human genetics: the changing politics of biotechnology governance in the European Union', *Health, Risk & Society*, 4 (3): 325–40.

Tesh, S. N. (2000) *Uncertain Hazards: environmental activists and scientific proof.* Ithaca, NY and London: Cornell University Press.

Touraine, A. (1981) *The Voice and the Eye: an analysis of social movements.* (A. Duff, trans.). Cambridge: Cambridge University Press.

—— (1983) 'Triumph or downfall of civil society', *Humanities in Review*, vol. 1. Cambridge: Cambridge University Press.

Turner, B. S. (2001) 'The erosion of citizenship', *British Journal of Sociology*, 52: 189–209.

Welsh, I. (2000) *Mobilising Modernity: the nuclear moment.* London: Routledge.

—— (2002) 'Where do movement frames come from? Insights from S26 and global "anti-capitalist" mobilisations', *Proceedings 8th Alternative Futures and Popular Protest Conference*, Vol. 2, Manchester: Manchester Metropolitan University.

—— (2006) 'Values, science and the EU: bio-technology and transatlantic relations', in I. Manners and S. Lucarelli (eds), *Values and Principles in EU Foreign Policy.* London: Routledge.

Welsh, I. and Evans, R. (1999) 'Xenotransplantation, risk, regulation and surveillance', *New Genetics and Society*, 18 (2/3): 197–217.

Welsh, I., Evans, R. and Plows, A. (2005) 'Another science for another world? Science and genomics at the London European Social Forum', Cardiff School of Social Sciences, Working Paper Series, No. 70. Available online at http://www.cardiff.ac.uk/schoolsanddivisions/academicschools/socsi/publications/working paperseries/index.html (accessed 21 July 2006).

Wynne, B. (1982) *Rationality and Ritual: the windscale inquiry and nuclear decisions in Britain.* Chalfont St Giles: BSHS.

—— (2005) 'Reflexing complexity: post-genomic knowledge and reductionist returns in public science', *Theory, Culture and Society*, 22 (5): 67–94.

Yearley, S. (1988) *Science, Technology & Social Change.* London: Routledge.

10 Genetics, gender and reproductive technologies in Latin America

Liliana Acero

Introduction

Challenging social and ethical issues are being confronted at the intersection of two major features of the contemporary world. First is the rapid emergence of new genetics and genomics knowledge and technologies. These pose especially difficult questions in the field of human reproduction – where developments such as in-vitro fertilization (IVF), screening for sex and other selection characteristics, and the use of stem cells are the focus of much controversy, and of efforts to establish public policies and professional practice (Annas 1998; Petersen and Bunton 2002; Davis 2001). Second, issues of international development, and specifically the 'health divide' between developed and developing countries, as well as the divides that exist within them (Daar *et al.* 2000; WHO 2002a). The two sets of issues relate, on the one hand, to international technology diffusion and management (WHO 2002b), and on the other, to population growth and reproductive rights (UNDP 2001; Galvez Perez and Matamala 2002; Petchesky and Corrêa 1994).

These are issues that have been typically studied in isolation, but the intersection of these two sets of features is profoundly important, as is apparent in European as well as in Latin American countries. Technologies have been developed that allow gametes, genes and embryos to be manipulated for research and fertilisation therapy, gene selection, enhancement or profit. If the technical and managerial skills are available, these technologies are relatively easy to transfer. In Latin American countries, the new technologies are being increasingly introduced to overcome infertility or the transmission of hereditary disorders. Research on, and applications of, new reproductive technologies (NRTs) question traditional norms and values (Luna 2003), giving rise to portrayals of the technologies as related to abortion or eugenics (Macklin 1999, 2000).

Numerous social and ethical concerns are associated with this biomedical research and its applications (Stein 2000; Council of Europe 1998; UNESCO 1997; Levine and Gorovitz with Gallagher 2000; CIOMS 2002; HFEA 1991). How these issues are confronted varies across countries, depending in part on cultural contexts, norms and values. In Latin America, problems associated with the use of NRTs are especially acute.

This chapter argues that lack of support for social research and governance frameworks on NRTs in Latin America can further intensify existing health divides, domestically and internationally. First, it briefly reviews the gender-aware international literature and discusses the main reasons for the scant evidence on Latin American NRTs. Second, it explores recent trends in local NRTs and shows how they question identity formation with specific relation to traditional norms and values. Third, it presents case-study results on the main socio-ethical dilemmas associated with their use in a context of limited regulatory frameworks and illustrates some transformations in local notions of pregnancy and motherhood. Finally, it concludes with policy recommendations for global and Latin American governance of NRTs.

Relevant international and regional studies

New reproductive technologies have been studied from a wide spectrum of approaches in cultural and social studies, sociology and anthropology, since the groundbreaking work of Rothman (1989), Corea (1986) and others. This has contributed to an established and wide-ranging debate on human reproduction that has been growing since the late 1970s. First, NRTs were analysed to explore different conflicts between traditional family values and choices of assisted conception (Ehrenreich and English 1978). Second, some studies addressed the many gender problems associated with the effects of the application of biomedical sciences, emphasising women's rights to control their bodies and exercise their autonomy in decision-making (O'Brien 1981). Third, much of this work set out to critique the commercialisation of procreation and also to problematise the controversial roles played by third-party donors and surrogate mothers in this context (Strathern 1993; Ragoné 1994; Rapp 1987). Fourth, the stigma attached to infertility, and the identification of ways to overcome it, were located within evolving social and gender constructs (Petchesky 1990). Fifth, many studies have been developed on the social implications of genetic testing, ultrasound techniques and the context of medicalised birth for the social representation of motherhood, foetuses and pregnancy (Weir 1996, 1998; Fox and Worts 1999). These studies also question how 'normalised' genetic screening could become potentially discriminatory, an argument also frequently raised by disability studies (see, e.g., Basen, Eichler and Lippman 1993). Sixth, feminist authors in particular have lately intensively addressed NRTs' global political implications and shown how these are rapidly reshaping and redefining the reproductive process (Ginsburg and Rapp 1995).

In the recent literature, only a few social studies have explored empirically social changes in the outcomes of assisted reproduction (exceptions include Stephen and McLean 1993; Cussins 1998) and of associated cultural transformations. The study of the perspectives, meanings and connections made by the public on these new technologies has been influential, due to the groundbreaking work undertaken by Edwards *et al.* (1993), Franklin (1997, 1998) and in Edwards's (2001) ongoing project on the public understandings of genetics. The authors show how nodes of meanings on genetics emerge and converge within culturally-determined understandings of kinship. This literature offers valuable insights for the study of public awareness on NRTs and the definition of policy.

There are rapid developments in scientific, ethical and legal discussions, public debate and political controversy regarding genetic innovations applicable to human reproduction and embryo screening (Marshall 2000; Galloux *et al.* 2002; Tong 2000). But positions taken by scholars tend to rest on a tenuous base of social science. In addition, while most studies do address the complexity of the social and human problems connected with innovations in procreation (Stacey 1992), and many show their effects on women (Ronchon Ford 2001), they overwhelmingly reflect the Euro-American cultural contexts where they were undertaken (with their specific meanings attached to the nuclear family, motherhood and kinship), even when they focus on cultural diversity within regions and countries (Ginsburg and Tsing 1990; for a critique see Purewal 2003).

By contrast, in Latin America there is a dearth of studies on the social consequences of the research on, and the use of, new reproductive technologies. Exceptions, such as Werneck *et al.* (2000), illustrate the particular way in which international differences in the socio-cultural and gender contexts where NRTs are applied affect the lives and decisions of local female end-users.

A few other studies address the specific bioethical questions that NRTs raise within the Latin America context. They usually emphasise the role of Catholic doctrine in shaping their development (Luna 2002; Acero 2003) or they quote this doctrine to support banning or very strict control of NRTs (Colombo 1999). A few studies (Alba Medrano 2002, Coe and Hanft 2001; Annas *et al.* 2002), very briefly explore the regional legal aspects related to NRTs, and whilst these offer useful descriptions of country-specific regulations and legal frameworks, they were not designed to analyse specific research questions.

There has been a stream of work on the biotechnology industry, usually driven by concerns about changes in innovation systems or economic performance, dealing mainly with genetically-modified crops, animal research genetics and biopharmaceuticals. However, these studies are carried out quite independently from the wider ethical and social concerns posed by genetic-based technologies and especially by reproductive technologies.[1]

This lack of evidence in the field partly reflects the positions adopted by local social scientists, the scientific community and government representatives on these new technologies. On the one hand, they tend to be mainly regarded as a First World topic by regional feminists and gender scholars, as well as international organisations supporting reproductive and women's health, social research and advocacy. The main argument is usually that: (a) they affect very few – and, almost exclusively, wealthy – women in the region; and, (b) more substantive women's health problems and inequalities should be the main topic for research and action. Governments tend to give priority to the reduction of maternal and child mortality/morbidity and other 'more pressing' regional health problems, problems they have agreed to counteract at various international government conferences such as the 1995 Beijing World Conference on Women. As a result, technologies and research are expanding in the region with little awareness amongst the general public, with practically no regulation or monitoring from governments or professional associations, and with little academic evidence to inform policy-making.

Given limited local resources, the directions taken and the priorities set regionally by mainstream health research and assistance cannot be radically questioned. However, continuing in this direction might further reproduce a health divide between developed and developing countries and increase internal social and gender inequalities. The new scientific and technological paradigm is at the forefront of world health research. For example, delays in developing substantive research on genomics and genetics and investing in training, competencies, genetic services and infrastructures mean that international inequalities increase and the health of local populations is negatively affected. Furthermore, poor Latin American women can become more prone to potential forms of 'genetics-related' abuse (for example, drug trials without consent, DNA sampling, removal of ova and tissues, trafficking of gametes, etc.), if evidence of local practices of NRTs is scant and societal debate and control scarce. This would eventually further increase domestic, international and gender inequalities.

Latin American discourse and practices

Throughout Latin America, double standards are applied to the use of embryos in research and treatment. In most countries, priority is given to protect the 'embryo's right to life'. The personhood of embryos from the zygote stage after conception becomes more relevant than women's needs, choices and rights, even when pregnancy might result in risks to the mother's health. Abortion is illegal in most countries and both practitioners and women undergoing abortion can be severely penalised and may face imprisonment.

This position towards embryos is held not only by the Catholic Church, but also by the medical community, and it is evident in prevailing regulations. However, there is a marked difference between voiced positions and real practice.

The World Health Organisation estimates that 21 per cent of maternal deaths related to pregnancy, childbirth and post-childbirth in Latin American countries are caused by complications from clandestine abortions, estimated to be in the order of four million a year (Alan Guttmacher Institute 1999). A substantive proportion of this number correspond to adolescent pregnancies.[2] Clandestine abortions are usually practised under extremely unsafe conditions. In some countries in the region[3] abortion is illegal in all circumstances; in others,[4] it is allowed in cases of rape, incest or when the life or health of the mother is severely threatened. Voluntary abortions (up to the eighth week of pregnancy) are only legal in Barbados, Cuba, Guyana and Puerto Rico.

Widely-held double standards result in a number of issues (Luna 2003). First, although not forbidden by law, there is a certain reluctance in some medical and scientific communities to freeze embryos. This is because embryos are considered persons. Second, most couples undergoing in-vitro fertilisation have to consent to donate their spare embryos, after a set time following the treatment, as embryos cannot be legally discarded. Third, the donation of eggs and embryos is frequently referred to as 'prenatal adoption', although it is not treated as a regular legal adoption. This usage is biologically confusing, and also places an extra emotional burden on women, parents and families. Women usually undergo several successive in-vitro fertilisation cycles, experience many pregnancy losses before any success, and often grieve over their miscarriages. The language of prenatal adoption can add a new stress to the already stressful process of in-vitro fertilisation.

Fourth, the use of pre-implantation diagnosis (PGD) to detect genetic disorders is usually available during in-vitro treatment. But it leads to the paradox that 'faulty' embryos can be detected but they cannot legally be discarded, though practitioners '*de facto*' have leverage to choose which embryos to implant. In some cases, fertility clinics encourage women to continue with their pregnancies. Finally, in Latin America in-vitro fertilisation treatment is allowed solely for married heterosexual couples and especially for younger women (under 35 years old), following mainstream religious opinion and social conventions. However, in Argentina, same-sex marriages have lately become legal and local women are having their first child much later in life, following worldwide trends to postpone marriage and pregnancy (Acero 1991).

In contrast, NRTs are expanding in the region, although only in some countries, such as Brazil and Chile, are there recently publicly-supported programmes of in-vitro fertilisation. Regulations are general and there is no national law or government monitoring of private fertility clinics. Actual practices tend to be informally guided by consensus documents produced by the medical and scientific communities, which are not binding. Usually, the practice of secrecy in egg, sperm and embryo donation is well established. This results in no follow-up of actual practices. Without such follow-up there is no evidence of how far laws and mores based on embryo personhood are really adhered to.

Latin American trends in NRTs

In 1984, the first baby was born from assisted conception in the region. Between 1991 and 1998, a total of 6,952 clinical pregnancies and 6,480 live births were reported by the Latin American Registry of Assisted Reproduction. These took place in ninety-three clinics in eleven different countries. Major contributions to in-vitro (IVF) and other forms of fertilisation were from Brazil (46.6 per cent of cases), Argentina (22.8 per cent) and Mexico (9.6 per cent), with Venezuela (5.8 per cent), Colombia (5.1 per cent) and Chile (5.0 per cent) showing similar rates of initiated cycles (Balmaceda *et al.* 2000).

Some of the main problems associated with the application of these techniques internationally are particularly acute in Latin America. These are mainly: (a) low success-rates – as low as a take-home-baby ratio of between 15 and 20 per cent, found by Franklin (1998) in the best clinics in the world. LARA (1998) reports an increase in birthrate for the region between 1990 and 1998 from 13.4 per cent to 19.0 per cent (pregnancy rates for the same period were 20.8 per cent and 27.8 per cent); (b) higher multi-gestation rates than global ones (30.6 per cent in 1998 for the region as against 28.1 per cent in 1990) and with a higher proportion of triplets and quadruplets births (20.6 per cent of twins and 7.5 per cent of triplets in 1998); and (c) an excessive amount of embryo-transfer per treatment cycle (3.2 the average embryo transfer in 1998, compared to Europe's maximum embryo transfer of two per cycle).

Also, multiple pregnancies increase the risk of stillbirth and prenatal mortality and morbidity because of the loss of weight associated with premature birth. In Latin America in 1998, stillbirth rates were 1.0 per cent from IVF and 1.3 per cent from ICSI technique (in-vitro cytoplasmatic sperm injection) (LARA 1998). Some evidence of higher risk of cerebral palsy (Stromberg *et al.* 2002 and Berg *et al.* 1999) among premature children, and of congenital malformations, genetic defects and tumours (Bonduelle *et al.* 1995; ESHRE 2000) in multi-gestations, has been found in European contexts, and has still to be further researched in Latin America.

Older ages of pregnancy tend to be associated with an increase in the rates of unsuccessful pregnancies, malformations and stillbirths from assisted conception. Between 1996 and 1998, LARA (1998) reports a relative increase in malformation rates among children from IVF (from 0.7 per cent to 2.0 per cent). It also shows that the age of female IVF patients increased between 1990 and 1998. In 1990, the proportions of women initiating treatment in different age cohorts was 66.5 per cent (< 35 years), 24.8 per cent (35–39 years), 8.7 per cent (> 39 years); in 1998, the proportions had changed to 50.4 per cent, 35.7 per cent and 13.9 per cent respectively.

Since the 1980s, Latin American NRTs have developed within a context of substantive gender inequalities. Assisted reproductive technologies only found a specific niche in the health services 'market' in Europe in the 1980s. Soon afterwards, exports of NRTs' medical tools and industrialised products to developing countries expanded (Ramírez 2003). Brazil was one of the Latin American countries most open to these imports. It promoted the training of local medical staff by foreign specialists, as well as the testing of experimental techniques domestically (Corrêa and Diniz 2000). At present, the majority of the Brazilian fertility clinics and hospitals are private (Corea 1996). It is estimated that two-thirds of Brazilian data related to assisted reproduction goes unreported within the country, as is the case in most of the region. In the other Latin American countries, clinics are massively concentrated in the capital cities and many times have doubled their number during the last decade.

In 1990, The Latin American Network on Assisted Reproduction (LARA) – a private initiative – was created to overcome the lack of information on outcomes from assisted reproduction, for inter-professional surveillance and exchange. It publishes periodic reports that evaluate data from fertility clinics in eleven countries in the region. However, there is no control, external to the profession, of the daily activities performed in these clinics or any reliable data on the number of frozen embryos in their sperm banks. And, there are virtually no available studies published or unpublished on the consequences of IVF treatments for the health of women and children.

The more traditional techniques of assisted reproduction (like artificial insemination) are applied together with complementary techniques, which are considered unsafe by international standards. These include high-ovulation protocols, with the use of recombinant follicle stimulating human hormone (FSH), which has been associated with epithelial ovarian cancer. Vayena *et al.* (2003) list six globally used techniques that should be considered only experimental.[5] There is evidence that some of them are used in Latin America, most specifically the ICSI treatments for male infertility which are routinely applied and highly recommended locally.

The cost of reproductive technologies varies widely between countries in the region, but it is generally very high. It can range from between US$ 2,500 and US$ 3,500 for each IVF attempt, and women regularly undergo at least three cycles before success.[6] However, there already exist viable low-cost protocols in assisted reproduction (Vayena, Rowe and Griffin 2003).

In Brazil, public health services began to offer assisted reproduction through public/private agreements. Local modern reproductive attitudes expanding into the public sector, exposed deep social contradictions. Diniz and Gonzalez Velez (2000) report that in Brazil, female patients in the public sector have either had a significant history of unsafe abortion that led them to infertility or had been prematurely sterilised.[7] Viable national legislation on NRTs has been discussed by the Congress in different countries. In Brazil and Chile, for example, law projects on assisted reproduction have been pending in Congress for almost a decade. During the scarce public debates, deep clashes have occurred between different professions and social groups. Feminist public positions are still scarcely represented in debates within Brazil, Chile and Argentina, and NRTs have not been systematically included in the agenda of the organised women's health movement.

Social, gender and ethical concerns

This section addresses some of the most relevant social, gender and ethical concerns in Latin American NRTs compared with those of developed countries: the treatment and research use of embryos, the process of informed consent, the disclosure of confidential information, and the provision of awareness to patients and the public.

Treatment and research use of embryos and the role of gamete/embryo donors

International concern at the risks to embryos and foetuses would seem irrelevant for Latin America, given the moral and legal status of embryos as persons. During my research, the use of spare ova/embryos in research and the discarding of 'abnormal' embryos were acknowledged, in spite of religious, legal and social conventions. For example, one fertility clinic in Argentina announces pre-implantation genetic diagnosis as follows:

> Transfer of an affected embryo is thus avoided, since only normal embryos are transferred. In this way, a couple or individuals with serious transmissible disorders avoid the risk of having affected offspring.

In addition, the consent form developed by the Latin American Network (Zegers-Hochschild and Pacheco 2001) includes a section on ovarian stimulation and the donation of ova to other patients. The female patient must make a choice between donation to other women, donation to the laboratory for 'biological trials' or for research, or elimination of the ova. In the case of donation for research, the patient is entitled to a consent form explaining: the nature of the research and whether ova will be exposed to fertilisation; the potential benefits of the activity for the patient or owner; the benefits for third parties; and the potential risks.

The source of donations is still an unresolved issue in Latin America. The voluntary donation of spare gametes/embryos between couples undergoing

IVF is reported as the source of many IVF treatments. Voluntary gamete donation is also frequently sought from close friends or relatives. The general open agreement in Latin America is that, in any case, it should not involve any form of payment. However, this raises a number of questions concerning the interests of the local poor. (If paid transactions of gametes/embryos were legalised, would this avoid any covert coercion or manipulation of the vulnerable poor?)

Screening of donors ranks high among worldwide concerns on NRTs, given the HIV/AIDS epidemic (Borrero 2003). In the past, sperm and eggs were not necessarily screened to standards currently considered acceptable, and these may still form part of local egg and sperm banks. Some sperm donors have been screened for infectious disease but not necessarily for hereditary disorders or general health status. Some local clinics advertise that they pursue the two first screens in their gamete banks, but not the third. Usually, screening relies heavily upon donors' voluntary verbal or written declarations, and this casts doubts about accuracy. Moreover, third-party egg donors are not regularly screened for general health status. Also, the sex-selection of couples' or donors' embryos, though outlawed in Latin America, may be secretly or orally advertised and practised, given scant regulations (similar to trends in other developing countries or minorities in developed countries (Purewal 2003).

The informed consent process

Sherwin (2000) shows how the type of informed consent regularly prac-tised is mainly related to a concept of individual free choice or consumer choice, which largely disregards the wider context in which it is exercised. It is equated to the exercise of rational preferences without interference or coercion – hardly the situation of most women in Latin America, given the extent to which gender influences medicalised birth options. Educational backgrounds, religious beliefs and social interactions also condition 'choices' and, in the Latin American context, women's autonomy presents a specific kind of vulnerability within the predominant constellation of relationships. This particular form of 'relational autonomy' is in turn both interpersonal and political, as can be exemplified during the informed consent process.

A standardised consent form booklet is available to all fertility clinics in LARA. It explains eight different aspects for which written consent is requested, and, for each stage, a form is signed by the couple and the doctor, following international practices. However, a number of flaws can be detected. This type of informed consent does not protect the patient's privacy, as forms are expected to be signed by both members of the couple, regardless of the quality of their relationship and of the potential influence of gender-constructs on the woman's decisions.

Further, the process is fragmented, with the patient acknowledging one step at a time and losing the general picture. The language in which the descriptions are made is far from colloquial, indeed almost technical, and assumes the reader has a fairly high level of formal schooling and can comfortably use abstract reasoning. And, for some of the steps, the information on risks and alternatives is insufficient. For example, the following paragraph in the booklet, relating ICSI procedures, illustrates the standard of text. After explaining that, as age increases some ova have more probability of presenting chromosomal abnormalities, it states:

> When more than one oocyte is fertilized, there will be more than one embryo. If more than one embryo is transferred, there is a higher probability for more than one to be normally formed and implanted. This is why when more embryos are transferred, the probability of pregnancy increases. However, it also increases the probability of multiple births.
>
> (Zegers-Hochschild and Pacheco 2001: 29 (my translation))

No other well-known risks of ICSI are mentioned, such as the high risk of congenital malformations due to specific manipulations, nor are doubts about the fertility of the male offspring conceived this way. Moreover, the entire booklet provides no counselling on the implications of, and arrangements for parenting in case of multiple births.

Individual fertility clinics decide unilaterally whether they give formal counselling before informed consent, and on how to structure it. Case material shows enormous disparities in counselling strategies. This reflects variations in the quality of counsellors' training in Latin America. Within counselling, adoption as an alternative choice is hardly discussed with clients, in spite of low success rates in treatments, relatively easy access to adoption and large numbers of children without parents throughout the region.

There is also widespread local debate on the efficacy of informed consent itself, reflecting wider global concerns about the validity of mainstream mechanisms. Analysing international health research, Lolas, for example, states that:

> Transcultural research simply means that researcher and participants come to the research with different cultural values and beliefs. The clash between world-views involves perceptions, forms of literacy, expectations and language.
>
> (Lolas 2000: 136)

Lolas recommends finding ways of promoting informed consent that take into account cultural, ideological, ethnic, gender and religious differences. He also advocates the development of bonds with the patients, based on consent dialogue, that would facilitate assessing their implicit and explicit beliefs. This strategy is aimed at counteracting the implicit subordination of the most vulnerable.

Record-keeping, health follow-ups and the disclosure of confidential information

The informed consent booklet analysed in the previous section does not refer to the situation of mothers, children or donors after treatments are completed. Information on patients and on spare embryos is kept for an average of four years. After that time, it is usually impossible to track ex-patients down, and/or spare embryos are not kept in banks. It also shows how little support is given to women and families post-pregnancy.

Insufficient or faulty record-keeping procedures interfere with follow-ups. In spite of LARA' s initiatives, standardised record-keeping is absent from many aspects of assisted reproduction. The concepts and categories through which data is collected and published are not clearly defined, making it very difficult to develop adequate social indicators. For example, the number of cycles initiated per woman cannot be easily calculated from published data. It is then not possible to base counselling on real research outcomes, i.e. from follow-up studies on IVF children and mothers, or to develop longitudinal studies on their health and psychological well-being. Moreover, access to specific records within LARA is largely limited to the participating clinics.

Cultural differences define notions of privacy in specific contexts. Extended families usually rely on the participation of other family members in the decision-making processes that surround natural pregnancy and motherhood (Acero 1991). Similar attitudes can be found in assisted conception. The stigma still attached to infertility – mainly among the poor – makes infertile couples and women more private in their decisions on assisted conception. However, it does not totally rule out key relatives' participation when couples are faced with critical decisions during infertility treatments.

Some studies show that sudden disclosure of their IVF origins to children tends to be highly detrimental (Hardy and Kuch 2003). They recommend that the process of disclosure be professionally guided. These studies also discourage withholding information on origins from children and show the negative consequences family secrets have upon their physical and psychological well-being. In Latin America, disclosure is largely decided by the parents on their own, an exception being the few Argentine fertility clinics that work with psychological support teams.

Provision of awareness to patients and the public

While in developed countries public enquiries and consultation on NRTs has been growing in the last decade, Latin America has only had sporadic surges of public debate. Media coverage of infertility, NRTs and contraception is limited, often due to Church pressures. Massive coverage occurs at specific times, related to a critical event, for example; in Brazil, during the Norplant contraceptive clinical trials; in Argentina, when a judge uni-laterally decided recently to prohibit family-planning activities in one of the country's provinces; in Chile, when the local Catholic Church inter-fered with an HIV/AIDS television campaign promoted by the government, and, for example, due to debates over the legalisation of the emergency pill. NRTs are even less discussed by the media.

Fertility and infertility form part of separate plans within health systems. They are not addressed by most reproductive health programmes, which tend to focus on sexual education and family planning. Thus, coherent national policies on reproduction are hard to develop. There are also lim-ited initiatives on patient advocacy and support groups on reproductive health, in particular on infertility and IVF. The latter are sometimes socially discouraged.

Scarce public resources have been geared to infertility prevention, as well as to research on its causes, frequently associated with sexually-transmitted diseases (STDs), and complications from unsafe clandestine abortions and occupational health hazards. For example, in Argentina, Chile and Brazil, regular screening does not usually scan for chlamydia, a well-known and usually invisible cause of inflammatory disorders in the Fallopian tubes which, if left unattended, can lead to female infertility. Given that difficult gender negotiations surround the use of male condoms, chlamydia has become an extremely generalised source of female infection, specially among vulnerable populations (Galvez Perez and Matamala 2002).

If this lack of public awareness continues, it would be extremely difficult to encourage the participation of an informed lay public in future govern-ing or oversight bodies for NRTs. In countries where democratic frame-works do not permeate society, only active citizen control can ensure the governance of confidential information. The participation of women's orga-nisations, health practitioners' associations and patients' support groups in NRT forums might be decisive for institutional accountability. Moreover, local women's organisations need explicitly to address the relation between genomics and society within their public agendas, to encourage female public awareness.

Changing notions of pregnancy and motherhood

Eichler (2001) shows that families, as contested political ground, have been defined historically in a number of different ways. Various dimensions of familial interaction (marital, procreative, emotional, sexual and so on) are subject to redefinition, given how NRTs influence changes in social relation-ships.[8] NRTs allow for the separation between the genetic and the gesta-tional mother, the inclusion – during pregnancy, of potential third parties as genetic or gestational substitutes (donors, surrogate mothers) and the retrieval of eggs for fertilisation from dead genetic and/or gestational mothers (includ-ing women kept on life support after death and who deliver babies through

caesarean section). These new genetic-based possibilities reframe local identities in a number of ways. For example, they mediate perspectives on kinship, interconnections between women, visions on the handicapped and,
most specifically, the notions of motherhood, pregnancy and family.

Whilst cultural specificities have been maintained, Latin America has not
been exempt from the reformulation of traditional kinship relations,
Women still tend to be devalued in the region if, after the age of 35, they
do not have children. Interviewees expressed that 'they feel sorry for them'
or that 'there is something very wrong with them'. And, it is frequently
taken for granted that lack of children is due to infertility. Werneck *et al.*
(2000) show how the word 'Yerma', meaning an arid desert (and the name
of the main character in a poem by Garcia Lorca), is popularly applied to
women who do not have children.

The need for approval, the loss of social identity and a sense of belonging is strongly felt by women who have made the choice not to have children as well as by those who are infertile.[9] Social pressure was reported by
our female interviewees as the second reason for initiating IVF treatment,
the first being the desire to have a biological child. Social conventions and
beliefs, impacted by generalised early religious training, present biological
motherhood as a 'natural' drive in women, and sometimes as 'God's
desire'. Fertility clinics use this type of approach to advertise their services.

Science and technology is positioned as a bridge between the infertile
woman and life itself. Social demand for the new techniques is portrayed
as 'developing beyond human control'. One fertility clinic in Argentina
markets innovation by showing how they 'invest in the emotional aspect of
assisted reproduction'.

> When we think about infertility, we give priority to the biological
> aspects. We know that the important technological advances at the
> service of assisted reproduction try to *correct or avoid flaws in
> women who can't get pregnant. Nevertheless, becoming parents and
> having a child goes far beyond body functions. ... It requires an
> emotional and affective disposition and patients frequently confront
> decision making over new issues. Current procedures propose differ-
> ent alternatives which the couple have to consider, avoiding pre-
> judices, ambivalences and questions.* At the same time, throughout
> the search for pregnancy, expectations, illusions and disillusions arise.
> *The rhythm of biological processes means following the ovulation
> cycles or follicular development times. These have a different time-
> table from emotional processes.*
>
> (my emphasis)

Infertility, in accordance with social conventions, is described as a 'flaw';
desire as the motive to have only *biological* children; parents-to-be are
reminded about the need for a positive emotional disposition to 'go beyond

their prejudices' to achieve success. Biology is alternatively and para-doxically portrayed as either autonomous of emotions and social norms or ruled by them.

This mixed approach towards assisted conception illustrates the equally mixed perceptions of new social and gender roles in these Latin American societies-in-transition. Psychologists dealing with IVF patients interviewed in Argentina and Chile reported that, while women are more likely to consider NRTs, shame, guilt and feelings of transgression may shape these choices which are seen as deviating from mainstream social norms.

Genetic screening has expanded even more than IVF in the region and poses a similar deconstruction of the intertext of pregnancy. Medicalised childbirth in the 1990s included regular ultrasounds and genetic screening for birth defects (amniocentesis and others), mainly for middle- and upper-class pregnant women over 35 years old. In the context of illegal and unsafe clandestine abortions, local women, more than those in developed countries, face 'their new reality as moral philosophers' and 'gatekeepers' of their children's health (Rapp 2000). They are responsible in a new way for key decisions involving future generations. Decisions on selective abortion – when embryos present disorders that might lead to severe handicap – become more complex in societies with illegal abortion, high levels of unemployment, low wages and working conditions. Decisions are further complicated when free or inexpensive care for special needs is severely limited and when urban environments are scarcely equipped to deal with disabilities. Some of our interviewees commented that the possibility of having a disabled child would lead them to consider clandestine abortion, in spite of risks, religious beliefs and moral remorse.

In summary, the rapid social changes produced by the new genetics within the ethical, socio-economic, and gender specificities of the Latin American context have created a great deal of ambiguity and ambivalence in the meanings attached to NRTs by women, patients, researchers and practitioners.

Concluding policy recommendations

The evidence presented supports the view that infertility treatments in Latin America should be regarded as part of reproductive rights, and that these treatments should be gradually included in mainstream public health coverage. By developing low-cost protocols, these treatments could be integrated through a quota system within the allocation of health resources. But before this type of policy can be efficiently and safely implemented, consistent national regulatory frameworks for assisted reproduction and research should be established. This could minimise growing risks of scattered practices and contradictory policies when these techniques become more popular. The diffusion of NRTs within Latin America has acute effects on the expansion of local stem cell research and gene therapy. Therefore, NRTs regulation may have an impact upon the whole field of human genetics positively, and help establish an adequate short-term institutional framework, based on accountability, transparency and citizen control.

Resources for infertility prevention should be substantively increased. General reproductive health programmes should deal jointly and consistently with fertility and infertility, contraception and assisted reproduction, in a manner that allows for coherent decision-making and suitable policy comparisons.

International agendas and lobbies should focus on discussing empirical evidence on NRTs in developing countries, and in Latin America in particular, where there is a scarcity of social science data on new trends. The recent globalisation of NRTs calls for ethically-sound international partnerships for the application of different techniques. The development of research studies that would provide results for evidence-based policy-making with a focus on developing countries should be a main priority for these international partnerships. An international consensus on basic principles towards the life sciences in their application to humans, one which takes account of different cultural practices, is needed if consistency in standard NRT practices and regulations is to be achieved.[10]

Notes

1 Exceptions are the Nuffield Council of Bioethics (1999) and Thomas (2003).
2 Brazilian adolescent births represent 26 per cent of total deliveries, the majority (42 per cent) from adolescents with a family income equivalent to US$ 80 (Rotania 2003).
3 Chile, Colombia, El Salvador, Honduras and the Dominican Republic.
4 Argentina, Brazil, Colombia, Venezuela, Costa Rica, Ecuador, Haiti, Jamaica, Nicaragua, Paraguay, Peru and Suriname.
5 Among them are: *in vitro* spermatogenesis, *in vitro* growth and maturation of oocytes, pregnancies with non-ejaculated sperm, spermatogonial stem-cell maturation and ICSI treatments.
6 Compared to between U$S 12,000 and U$S 15,000 per treatment cycle in the USA, and an average five cyles for a successful birth; reported by Rapp (2000) and others.
7 In Brazil, surgical sterilisation is the first method of contraception for women between 15 and 49 years old.
8 She also considers full, partial, exclusive and non-exclusive parenting and finds twenty-five different types of mothers and nine types of fathers with NRTs.
9 For similar findings see, the Warnock Report (Warnock 1985) and Franklin (1997).
10 See the proposals of UNESCO's Division of Ethics of Science and Technology, e.g. UNESCO (2004), and relating reproductive cloning initiatives such as those of UNESCO's Intergovernmental Bioethics Committee since 2001, and those of the General Assembly of United Nations in March 2005.

References

Acero, L. (1991) *Textile Workers in Brazil and Argentina: work and household behaviour by gender and age.* Japan: United Nations University Press.

—— (2003) 'New reproductive technologies and gender: key concerns for Latin America', paper presented at the UNESCO-Carleton University Panel on the Life Sciences, November. Ottawa (unpublished observations).

Alan Guttmacher Institute (1999) *Sharing Responsibility: women, society and abortion worldwide: a special report.* Available online at http://www.guttmacher. org (accessed 24 July 2006).

Alba Medrano, Marcia Muñoz de (ed.) (2000) *Reflexiones en Torno al Derecho Genómico.* Mexico: Universidad Autónoma de México, Instituto de Investigaciones Jurídicas.

—— (2002) 'Aspectos sobre la regulación del genoma humano en México' (Considerations on the regulation of the human genome in Mexico), in M. Muñoz de Alba Medrano (ed.), *Reflexiones en torno al derecho genómico* (Reflections on genomic law). Mexico: UNAM, Instituto de Investigaciones Jurídicas.

Annas, G. (1998) *Some Choice, Law, Medicine and the Market.* Oxford: Oxford University Press.

Annas, G., Andrews, L. and Isasi, I. (2002) 'Protecting the endangered human: toward an international treaty prohibiting cloning and inheritable alterations', *American Journal of Law and Medicine*, 28: (1 and 2): 151–78.

Balmaceda, J., Galdames, V. and Zegers-Hochschild, F. (2000) *Registro Latinoamericano de Reproducción Asistida 2000.* Colombia: Red Latinoamericana de Reproducción Asistida.

Basen, G., Eichler, M. and Lippman, A. (eds) (1993) *Misconceptions: the social construction of choice and the new reproductive technologies*, Vols 1 and 2. Quebec: Voyageur Publishing.

Berg, T., Erikson, A., Hillensjo, T., Nygren, K. G. and Wennerholm, U. B. (1999) 'Deliveries and children born after in vitro fertilization in Sweden 1982-1995: a retrospective cohort study', *Lancet*, 354: 1579–85.

Bonduelle, M., Legein, J., Derde, M. P., Buysse, A., Schietecatte, J., Wisanto, A., Devroey, P. van Steirteghem, A. and Liebaers, I. (1995) 'Comparative follow-up study of 130 children born after ICI and 130 children born after IVF', *Human Reproduction*, 10: 3327–31.

Borrero, C. (2003) 'Gamete and embryo donation', in E. Vayena, P. Rowe and D. Griffin (eds), *Current practices and controversies in assisted reproduction: WHO report on a meeting on Medical, ethical and social aspects of assisted reproduction.* Geneva17–21 September 2001. Geneva: WHO.

CIOMS (2002) *International ethical guidelines for biomedical research involving human subjects.* Geneva: CIOMS.

Coe, G. and Hanft, R. (2001) 'The use of technologies in the healthcare of women: a review of the literature', in E. Gomez (ed.), *Gender, Women and Health in the Americas. PAHO Scientific Publications.* Washington: PAHO. 541: 195–207.

Colombo, R. (1999) 'La Naturaleza y el estatuto del embrión', *Revista Humanitas*, 16: 46–59.

Corea, G. (1986) *The Mother Machine: reproductive technologies from artificial insemination to artificial wombs.* New York: Harper & Rowe.

—— (1996) 'Os riscos da Fertilização in vitro', in L. Scavone (org.), *Tecnologias Reprodutivas: gênero eciência.* São Paulo: Editora da Universidade Estadual Paulista.

Corrêa, M. and Diniz, D. (2000) 'Novas Tecnologias Reprodutivas no Brasil: um debate à espera de Regulação', in F. Carneiro and M. C. Emerick (eds), *A Ética* eo *Debate Jurídico sobre Acesso e Uso do Genoma Humano*. Rio de Janheiro: Fiocruz.

Council of Europe (1998) *Convention of Human Rights and Biomedicine*, Luxembourg: Council of Europe.

Cussins, C. (1998) 'Producing reproduction: techniques of normalization and naturalization in fertility clinics', in S. Franklin and H. Ragoné (eds), *Reproducing Reproduction: kinship, power and technological innovation*. Philadelphia, PA: University of Pennsylvania Press.

Daar, A. S., Thorsteinsdottir, H., Martin, D. K., Smith, A. C., Nast, S. and Singer, P. A. (2000) 'Top ten biotechnologies for improving health in developing countries', *Nature Genetics*, 32 (2): 229–32.

Davis, D (2001) *Genetic Dilemmas: reproductive technology, parental choices and children's futures*. London: Routledge.

Diniz, D. (2002) 'Questões da Reprodução Humana (RHA e Genética)', in Rede Nacional Feminista de Saúde e Direitos Sexuais e Reprodutivos, *O feminismo eo SUS: as mulheres eo controle social*. São Paulo: RNFSDSR.

Diniz, D. and Gonzalez Velez, A. (2000) 'Feminist bioethics: the emergence of the oppressed', in R. Tong (ed.), *Globalizing Feminist Bioethics: crosscultural perspectives*. Boulder, CO: Westview Press.

Edwards, J. (2001) 'Public understanding of genetics: a cross-cultural study of the relationship between the new genetics and social identity: a project under the European Commission's Fifth Framework Programme', Manchester: Dept. of Social Anthropology, The University of Manchester (Unpublished observations).

Edwards, J., Hirsch, E., Price, F. and Strathern, M. (1993) *Technologies of Procreation: kinship in the age of assisted conception*. Manchester: Manchester University Press.

Ehrenreich, B. and English, D. (1978) *For her own Good: 150 years of the experts' advice to women*. New York: Doubleday.

Eichler, M. (2001) 'Biases in family literature', in M. Baker (ed.), *Families. Changing Trends in Canada*, 4th edition. New York: McGraw Hill

ESHRE Capri Workshop Group (2000) 'Multiple gestation pregnancy', *Human Reproduction*, 15: 1856–64.

Fox, B. and Worts, D. (1999) 'Revisiting the critique of medicalized childbirth: a contribution to the Sociology of Birth', *Gender and Society*, 13 (3): 326–46.

Franklin, S. (1997) *Embodied Progress: a cultural account of assisted conception*. London: Routledge.

—— (1998) 'Making miracles: Scientific progress and the facts of life', in S. Franklin and H. Ragoné (eds), *Reproducing Reproduction: kinship, power and technological innovation*. Philadelphia, PA: University of Pennsylvania Press

Franklin, S. and Ragoné, H. (1998) (eds) *Reproducing Reproduction: kinship, power and technological innovation*. Philadelphia, PA: University of Pennsylvania Press.

Galloux, J.-C., Mortensen, A., de Cheveigne, S., Allansdottir, A., Chatjouli, A. and Sakellaris, G. (2002) 'Institutions of Bioethics', in M. Bauer and Gaskell (eds), *Biotechnology: The making of a global controversy*. London: Cambridge University Press

Galvez Perez, T. and Matamala, M (2002) 'La economia de la salud yel género en la reforma de salud', paper presented at the Pan American Health Organization International Conference on Gender, Equity and Health Reform in Santiago, Chile, 10–12 April.

Ginsburg, F. and Rapp, R. (eds) (1995) *Conceiving the New World Order: the global politics of reproduction*. Berkeley and Los Angeles, CA: University of California Press.

Ginsburg, F. and Tsing, A. (eds) (1990) *Uncertain Terms: negotiating gender in American culture*. Boston, MA: Beacon Press.

Hardy, E. and Kuch, M. (2003) 'Gender, infertility and art', in. E. Vayena, P. Rowe and D. Griffin (eds), *Current Practices and Controversies in Assisted Reproduction: WHO report on a meeting on medical, ethical and social aspects of assisted reproduction*. Geneva 17–21 September 2001. Geneva: WHO.

Human Fertilization and Embryology Authority (HFEA) (1991) *Code of Practice: explanation*. London: HFEA.

Latin American Network of Assisted Reproduction (LARA) (1998) *Registro Latinoamericano de Reproducción Asistida*. Colombia: LARA.

Lolas, F. (2000) 'Intercultural communication and informed consent: commentary on (i) cultural influences and communication', in R. Levine and S. Gorovitz, with J. Gallagher, *Biomedical research ethics: updating international guidelines, a consultation*, Council for International Organisations of Medical Sciences. Geneva: CIOMS.

Luna, F. (2002) 'Commentary on reproductive biology and technology', in R. Levine and S. Gorovitz, with J. Gallagher, *Biomedical Research Ethics: updating international guidelines, a consultation*, Council for International Organisations of Medical Sciences. Geneva: CIOMS.

—— (2003) 'Assisted reproduction in Latin America: some ethical and socio-cultural issues', in. E. Vayena, P. Rowe and D. Griffin (eds), *Current Practices and Controversies in Assisted Reproduction: WHO report on a meeting on medical, ethical and social aspects of assisted reproduction*. Geneva 17–21 September 2001. Geneva: WHO.

Macklin, R. (1999) 'Is ethics universal? Gender, science and culture', in N. King, G. E. Henderson and J. Stein (eds), *Beyond Regulations: ethics in human subjects research*. Chapel Hill, NC and London: The University of North Carolina Press.

—— (2000) 'Reproductive biology and technology', in R. Levine and S. Gorovitz with J. Gallagher, *Biomedical Research Ethics: updating international guidelines, a consultation*, Council for International Organisations of Medical Sciences. Geneva: CIOMS. 208–26.

Marshall, P. (2000) 'Informed consent in international health research', in R. Levine and S. Gorovitz, with J. Gallagher, *Biomedical Research Ethics: updating international guidelines, a consultation*, Council for International Organisations of Medical Sciences. Geneva: CIOMS.

McNeil, M., Varcoe, I. and Yearley, S. (eds) (1990) *The New Reproductive Technologies*. London: Macmillan.

Nuffield Council of Bioethics (1999) The ethics of clinical research in developing countries: a discussion paper. London: n.p.

O'Brien, M. (1981) *The Politics of Reproduction*. London: Routledge and Kegan Paul.

Petchesky, R. (1990) *Abortion and Women's Choice: the state, sexuality and reproductive freedom*. Boston, MA: Northeastern University Press.

Petchesky, R. and Corrêa, S. (1994) 'Reproductive and sexual rights: a feminist perspective', in *Population Policies Reconsidered: health, empowerment and rights*. New York: Harvard University Press.

Petersen, A. and Bunton, R. (2002) *The New Genetics and the Public's Health*. London: Routledge.

Purewal, N. (2003) *Mothering Instincts: the ultrasound scan, sex selection and the politics of choice*, (unpublished observations), University of Manchester, Department of Sociology.

Ragoné, H. (1994) *Surrogate Motherhood: conception in the heart*. Boulder, CO and London: Westview Press.

Ramírez, M. (2003) *Novas Tecnologías Reprodutivas Conceptivas: fabricando avida, fabricando o futuro*, unpublished doctoral thesis, São Paulo: Universidade Estadual de Campinas, Instituto de Filosofia e Ciências Humanas.

Rapp, R. (1987) 'Moral pioneers: women, men and fetuses on a frontier of reproductive technology', *Women and Health*, 13(1–2): 101–16.

—— (2000) *Testing Women, Testing the Fetus: the social impact of amniocen thesis in America*. New York: Routledge.

Ronchon Ford, A. (2001) 'Biotechnology and the new genetics: what it means for women's health', paper prepared for the Working Group on Women's Health and the New Genetics, University of York and The Canadian Women's Health Network, Toronto, February.

Rotania, A. (2003) 'New contraception and genetic reproductive technologies: challenges, limits and perspectives of thought and action', paper presented at the Working Conference on the Challenges of the New Human Genetic Technologies: Within and beyond the limits of human nature. Berlin, 12–15 October.

Rothman, B. (1989) *Recreating Motherhood: ideology and technology in a patriarchal society*. New York: Norton.

Sherwin, S. (2000) 'Normalizing reproductive technologies and the implications for autonomy', in R. Tong (ed.), *Globalizing Feminist Bioethics: crosscultural perspectives*. Boulder, CO: Westview Press

Stacey, M. (ed.) (1992) *Changing Human Reproduction: social sciences perspectives*. London: Sage.

Stein, J. (ed.) (2000) *Beyond regulations: ethics in human subjects' research*. Chapel Hill, NC and London: The University of North Carolina Press.

Stephen, T. and McLean, J. (1993) *Survey of Canadian Fertility Programs*, paper presented to the Canadian Royal Commission on New Reproductive Technologies, Ottawa.

Strathern, M. (1993) *Reproducing the Future: anthropology, kinship and the new reproductive technologies*. Manchester: Manchester University Press.

Stromberg, B., Dahlquist, G., Ericson, A., Finnstrom, O., Koster, M. and Stjernqvist, K. (2002) 'Neurological sequelae in children born after in-vitro fertilization', *Lancet*, 359: 461–5.

Thomas, S. (2003) 'Critical issues pertaining to the gender dimension of biotechnology policy', paper presented to the Gender Advisory Board, United Nations Commission on Science and Technology for Development, Geneva, July.

UNDP (2001) *Human Development Report 2001: making new technologies work for human development*. New York: Oxford University Press.

UNESCO (1997) *Universal Declaration on the Human Genome and Human Rights*, Governmental Committee Meeting. UNESCO, BIO 97, Paris, Conf.201/5.

—— (2004) *National Legislation Concerning Human Reproduction and Therapeutic Cloning*, Division of Ethics of Science and Technology. UNESCO. Paris, April.

Warnock, M. (1985) *A Question of Life*. Oxford: Basil Blackwell.

Weir, L. (1996) 'Recent developments in the governance of pregnancy', *Economy and Society*, 25 (3): 372–92.

—— (1998) 'Cultural intertexts and scientific rationality: the case of pregnancy ultrasound', *Economy and Society*, 27 (2 and 3): 249–58.

Werneck, J., Carneiro, F., Rotania, A. A., Holmes, H. B. and Rorty, M. R. (2000) 'Autonomy and procreation: Brazilian feminist analyses', in R. Tong (ed.), *Globalizing Feminist Bioethics: crosscultural perspectives*. Boulder, CO: Westview Press.

WHO (2002a) *Collaboration in Medical Genetics*. A Report on a WHO meeting. Toronto, April 9–10.

—— (2002b) *Genetics and World Health*. The Advisory Committee on Health Research. Geneva: WHO.

Zegers-Hochschild, F. (2003) 'The spread of new reproductive technologies in Latin America', in. E. Vayena, P. Rowe and D. Griffin (eds), *Current Practices and Controversies in Assisted Reproduction: WHO report on a meeting on medical, ethical and social aspects of assisted reproduction*. Geneva 17–21 September 2001. Geneva: WHO.

Zegers-Hochschild, F. and Pacheco, I. (eds) (2001) *Red Latinoamericana de Reproducción asistida, Formulario de educación y consentimiento en procedimientos de reproducción asistida*, September. Colombia: LARA.

11 Genomics, social formations and subjectivity

Priya Venkatesan

Genomics has enormous potential for changing the way in which bio-medical scientific research is conducted. By simply arraying an RNA sample of a cancer patient on a microarray chip and comparing it with that of normal patients, one can potentially diagnose and administer treatment on the basis of determining which genes are expressed. Genes implicated in genetic disorders can be localised by virtue of information garnered from the Human Genome Project and used expressly for the purposes of gene therapy. Functional genomics studies facilitate the methods used to assign function to particular genes and further advance efforts to characterise genes. In short, a revolution has occurred in research *vis-à-vis* the emergence of genomics.

While most of the technology of genomics occurs in the laboratory, its effects have far-reaching implications for society, not only in the arena of medicine. In this chapter, I explore how social identity and cultural discourse are ultimately affected by the technological advancements of genomics. The teleology of genomics would be defined by the characterisation of everyone by their genetic make-up. This definition would translate into new social formations based on the genetic composition of a person. A new preconception of the subject would emerge and one's subjectivity would rely on scientific parameters rather than metaphysical attributes. Philosophy, once the origin of wisdom of the individual and his/her relation to society, would be replaced by molecular science, now the progenitor of a new designation of self. Concomitantly, an intellectual displacement of the human sciences would occur in terms of the insight it offers into the representation of the self. I would like to address how this process occurs. While I am not arguing that an extreme science-fiction scenario such as that depicted in the postmodern film *Gattaca* would occur, nevertheless the site of subjectivity would shift from the whole self to the gene.

Michel Foucault radically revised the concept of subjectivity; through his analysis of texts of ancient Greece and Rome, he argued for subjectivity as truth about oneself and elaborated on the art of ethics as self-mastery *vis-à-vis* the subject's position in the world. For Foucault the process of subjectivisation was not just a manifestation of individual introspection but of discovering self by its production through practices. The question of self and identity is not just a question of a human individual's attempt to discover who one is, but of external forces which make the self and are folded in the becoming of a human being. These external forces are integrated to build a self.

It is this delineation of the process of subjectivity concerning the Foucauldian method that forms my starting point on the sociological and cultural role that genomics plays in the organisation of social formations and the elements of discourse in contemporary culture. Under the same scope, the innovation of genomics moves from exemplifying scientific advancement to becoming a social object and is thereby transformed into an external force that shapes the way we view ourselves and our role in society. (In fact a colour booklet describing the science behind the Human Genome Project and endorsed by the Department of Energy, called *To Know Ourselves*, makes explicit reference to the role of subjectivity in genomics.)

In addition to changing radically the biological perspective from which we view gene function and disease, advances in genomics have made possible a new way of defining our subjectivity and identity through the lenses of genes, gene function and proteins. Technology derived from the Human Genome Project, and the scientific techniques that have benefited from it, have made possible the advanced mapping of genes on chromosomes, the characterisation of chromosomal changes in disease, and gene expression patterns during development and differentiation. These technical apparatuses have allowed for novel definitions of subjectivity based on the ability of these technologies to target variation and individuality. These technologies have been used to determine individual patterns in gene expressions between individuals. In other words, human uniqueness may be tantamount to genetic uniqueness, and the capacity to represent genetic uniqueness is further aided by genomics. To highlight and discuss these technologies in the context of what Paul Rabinow terms biosociality – that is, the collective effect that genomics has on social organisation and function – is to arrive at a new understanding of subjectivity approached from the perspective of molecular science (Rabinow 1996).

Advances in determining the genetic distinctions between disease and non-disease, between differences in drug responses and between good and bad prognosis, will ultimately affect the type of social formations and social forums that society engages in, and, simultaneously, an individual's preconception of himself or herself. Paradoxically, while these technologies emphasise the individual's uniqueness through genetic criteria, they illustrate, through their initial utilisation in diagnosis, prognosis and treatment of disease to their ultimate realisation in the categorisation of individuals, the process of subjectivisation, i.e. the transformation from personhood to subject, the move from uniqueness and distinctiveness of the individual to the subordination to the data of the patient. They exemplify the Foucauldian forces of exteriority at work in a 'society of genomics'.

The concept of identities refers to the dynamic making of selves in situations and contexts. Identity and the related concept of subjectivity have been written about from many different perspectives. These include psychoanalytic, Bakhtinian, Foucauldian and other poststructuralist approaches. One of the leading research centres which focuses on identity and the formation of the subject-citizen in the context of science is the Centre for Citizenship, Identity and Governance (CCIG). It was established in 2002–3, and has undertaken research on identity formation from a number of theoretical perspectives, including the effects of macro-social changes on identities, the role of the relationship in the making of the self, and the multiplicity and coherence in the organisation of contemporary identity configurations. These more theoretical concerns have practical implications in assessing changes in power and authority relations, effects on the regulation of conduct and moral subjectivity, changes in the expression of class, religious, ethnic and gender identities, and their effects on social structures such as employment, the church and the family (CCIG mission statement). CCIG researchers raise the issue that, if identity is understood in a psycho-social way, methods will need to be consistent with that approach.

This chapter will address methodologically how subjectivity is affected by the technology of genomics through Foucault's paradigms. My paradigm relies on Foucault's conceptualisation of how exterior forces are pivotal in the formation of self and the individual: that is, subjectivity. Foucault reorients research away from the ways in which scientific objects are constituted and towards the ways in which human beings are constituted as subjects of knowledge, in so far as they themselves become objects of knowledge and receive moral and psychological identities through scientific discourse (Best 1995: 91). In Foucault's words, 'While historians of science in France were interested essentially in the problem of how a scientific object is constituted, the question I ask myself was this: how is it that the human subject took itself as the object of possible knowledge? Through what form of rationality and historical conditions? And finally at what price?' (Foucault 1985: 29–30).

> How was the subject established, at different moments and in different institutional contexts, as a possible, desirable, or even indispensable object of knowledge? How were the experience that one may have of oneself and the knowledge that one forms of oneself organized according to certain schemes? How were these schemes defined, valorized, recommended, imposed? *It is clear that neither the recourse to an original experience nor the study of the philosophical theories of the soul, the passions or the body can serve as the axis in such an investigation.* The guiding thread that seems the most useful for this inquiry is constituted by what one might call the 'techniques of the self,' which is to say, the procedures, which no doubt exist in

every civilization, suggested or prescribed to individuals in order to determine their identity, through relations of self-mastery or self knowledge ... *It is amatter of the formation of the self through techniques of living, not of repression through prohibition and law.*

(Foucault 1985: 87–9; italics mine)

In this context, subjectivity is the province of self-generated proscriptions rather than individual introspection. Here, Foucault's citations attribute the subject's identity to the 'techniques of the self'. In turn, the natural uniqueness of each individual's genome has become an important issue for legal practice and human self-understanding, going so far as to implicitly define humanity, individuality and personhood (Hauskeller 2004).

These issues can be illustrated from a series of published studies in recent genomic science. Whitney *et al.* (2003) discuss and illustrate interindividual variation in peripheral blood cells, identified through microarray analysis. According to the authors, these data help to define human individuality and provide a database with which disease-associated gene expression patterns can be compared. The paper presents data as an extension of the numerous studies that have:

Described efforts to map and characterize variations in human gene expression patterns associated with differences in cell and tissue type, physiological processes, and disease ... The extent, nature and sources of variation in gene expression among [individuals] is a fundamental aspect of human biology. Further investigations of human gene expression associated with disease, and their potential application to detection and diagnosis, will depend on an understanding of their normal variation within and between individuals, over time, and with age, gender and other aspects of the human condition.

(Whitney *et al.* 2003).

The data reveal evidence of distinct patterns of interindividual variation and that some features of variation in expression patterns were reflective of genetic uniqueness. The authors conclude by terming the results a 'genome-scale molecular portrait of healthy human tissue'. This 'molecular portrait' itself is a new parameter for subjectivity, for a portrait, in its metaphorical sense, remains a telling reference to the self, or the image of the self in this case. The fact that the 'portrait' is described as molecular is an indication of the implications of genetics for subjectivity.

My second example derives from the work of Dumur *et al.* (2003). Their paper illustrates the molecular phenomenon of the loss of heterozygosity, which is considered a marker for tumour progression. Dumur *et al.* (2003) describe 'genome-wide detection of LOH in prostate cancer using human SNP microarray technology', loss of heterozygosity, or more frequently-termed LOH, has been localised on chromosomal regions using SNP (single nucleotide polymorphism) microarray technology in prostate cancer. A single nucleotide polymorphism is a unique nucleotide that exists in an individual's genome. The technical innovation here is the use of this uniqueness, as represented by SNPs, to identify whether certain alleles in prostate cancer patients lose their heterozygous nature. (This transformation of alleles from heterozygous to homozygous is an indication of the progression of many human cancers.) According to the authors, the LOH analysis was based on comparison of the genotypes from both the tumour and the normal samples from the same individual. At each locus, the genotypes were compared to determine allelic imbalance or LOH, retention of heterozygosity, or neither.

The technology of the Human Genome Project has made possible the cataloguing of human SNPs on a microarray. Through the use of this technology to detect LOH, as demonstrated by Dumur *et al.*, genetic individuality and the variation due to SNPs become prognostic and diagnostic indicators of disease, in this case prostate cancer. Because of the SNP chip microarray, chromosomal regions harbouring candidate tumour suppressor genes implicated in human cancers can be more easily identified, since these regions demonstrate high rate of loss of genetic material and frequently contain tumour suppressor genes. Therefore, as LOHs are identified on a large scale, the propensity for cancer in an individual is more easily determined. This type of genetic uniqueness, as illustrated by LOH, may be a potential indicator of how new social organisations based on genetic determinants, that is, those with and without LOHs, can come to fruition. By becoming aware of one's genetic disposition to cancer, an individual's notion of self may be ultimately determined by his or her own cognizance of potentially acquiring a disease. While this discussion remains in the sphere of 'potentialities', a definitive possibility remains that the parameters of subjectivity may be radically altered by this technology.

A further example is provided by the work of Wen *et al.* (1998), who generated a temporal map of gene expression during central nervous system development. The element of time was introduced into gene expression profiles. The authors attempted to understand possible functional relationships between gene families by examining their patterns of expression over the course of development. In this instance, the data they present provides a 'temporal gene expression "fingerprint" of spinal cord development based on major families of inter- and intra-signaling genes' (Wen *et al.* 1998). A fundamental aspect of this functional genomics is a straightforward cataloguing of gene expression in different species and tissues. This research is illustrated with gene expression waves representing normalised trajectories of patterns and clustering them in groups depending on their temporal expression. These waves represent a unique, innovative way to illustrate cell development (from proliferation to differentiation in the CNS). They represent 'the systematic measurement of multiple gene expression time series, producing a temporal map of developmental gene expression'.

Through the accommodation of temporality into the parameter of gene expression, the factor of time is introduced into the conceptual terrain of genetic uniqueness. As patterns of gene expression in development are revealed, individuality and variation are now functions of time.

These results, according to the authors, suggest functional relationships among genes fluctuating in parallel. These genes occur in clusters according to their class and function. Furthermore, the concepts and data analysis discussed by Wen *et al. may* be useful in objectively identifying coherent patterns and sequences of events in the complex genetic signalling network of development. As genes can be classified according to their function in terms of their developmental pattern, genetic uniqueness can be further characterised in terms of development. Since these studies are aimed at the elucidation of complex developmental and degenerative disorder, a gene expression wave is another approach to distinguishing between the healthy and the diseased.

As these patterns of temporal gene expression concretely differ in their depict, (one set of waves will have different trajectories, colours and patterns from another), an individual's waves will concretely represent a unique developmental pattern. These pictures of gene expression waves and the cataloguing of developmental gene patterns depicted could be understood as pictures of subjects, pictures with which those involved in scientific and clinical work and its objects have to engage. Similar to gene expression profiling through microarrays and the chromosomal instability of LOH, the temporality of gene expression waves is a point of subjectivisation for the subject, from the perspective of the individual. Each instance of time is a moment when the subject is represented; gene expression waves are the conceptualisation of the process of subjectivity. The implications for subject formation are inherent in the exploitation of these data for further characterising variation in development and the cataloguing of that variation into discrete tools for evaluating normality.

It is not simply that the data from these technologies themselves have enormous impact on subjectivity and social organisation; but the methods used to make sense of those data are now progenitors of expressions of individuality and of the subject. Self-organising maps, a mathematical tool that recognises certain biological features of data, were applied to red blood cell differentiation in order to determine blocks in the developmental programme that likely underlie the pathogenesis of leukaemia (Tamayo *et al.* 1999). According to the authors, self-organising maps recognise and classify features in complex, multi-dimensional data. This tool has been packaged in a publicly available form called GENECLUSTER. Tamayo *et al.* assayed the expression patterns of some 6,000 human genes, and used GENECLUSTER to 'organize the genes into biologically relevant clusters that suggest novel hypotheses about, [in this case], hematopoietic differentiation – for example, highlighting certain genes and pathways involved in differentiation therapy used in treatment of [leukemia]'.

Self-organising maps, like hierarchical clustering, are an extension of the scientific methods used to amass data and to produce results, since they are particularly useful for analysing gene expression patterns and exposing fundamental patterns in those data. In this study, the maps revealed clusters of genes in certain myelocytic cell lines that were responsible for differentiation of haematopoietic cells. As diseased cell lineages were the objects of study, self-organising maps distinguish diseased states and configure subjectivity in distinctive ways. By representing gene expression patterns uniquely, these maps are illustrations of individuality and uniqueness. They designate a certain type of variability. However, much like the other technical representations, they inure the individual to the category of subject as patient. The power of this technology would further intensify this process.

Microarrays are an interesting, innovative approach to understanding how genetics could determine subjectivity, especially in terms of implications for genetic profiling, and form a topic in themselves. In general, it would be more economical to mass-produce microarrays printed with DNA from normal individuals.[1] Doctors could purchase these arrays and probe them with labelled cDNA from cancer patients to see how they differ from non-cancer expression levels. This type of approach is commonly being used now to define the genes that are differentially expressed in different types of cancer in order to further define the function of those gene products *in vivo*. It is quite reasonable that, in the future, this method could be used as a diagnostic approach, either once cancer has been detected, or beforehand, to determine the need for preventive measures (and to identify which measures could be taken). However, genetic profiling of an individual without cancer is not likely to be very predictive, since environmental factors play a large role in the development of many types of cancer. And the identification of factors that point towards the likely development of a cancer, such as a genetic predisposition for breast cancer, does not necessarily mean that the patient will develop cancer, just that they are more likely to.

The organising potential of the technology from the Human Genome Project is ultimately realised in the field of pharmacogenomics, which is a way of characterising interindividual differences to drug responses based on knowledge of an individual's genetic polymorphisms. According to Evans and Johnson (2001), for example, the ultimate goal is to provide new strategies for optimising drug therapy based on each patient's genetic determinants of drug efficacy and toxicity. The vision is that, in the future, authorised clinicians will be able to access a secure database in which their patients' genetic polymorphisms will have been recorded, as they are determined for specific classes of medications based on their illnesses. Technology will ultimately make it possible to perform a genome-wide scan for polymorphisms that are associated with disease risk or drug response, such that these data will be determined *a priori* and thus will be available to clinicians for preventive health and prospective treatment decisions (Evans and Johnson 2001). Genetic uniqueness can now be methodologically organised under technical supervision for medical purposes. In this light, the authors continue:

> It is well recognized that most medications exhibit wide interpatient variability in their efficacy and toxicity. For many medications, these interindividual differences are due in part to polymorphisms in genes encoding drug metabolizing enzymes, drug transporters, drug targets. Pharmacogenomics is a burgeoning field aimed at elucidating the genetic basis for differences in drug efficacy and toxicity, and it uses genome-wide approaches to identify the network of genes that govern an individual's responses to drug therapy.
>
> (Evans and Johnson 2001: 9)

The purported objective of pharmacogenomics is to achieve optimal drug therapy:

> Pharmacogenomics aims to elucidate the network of genes that determine the efficacy and toxicity of specific medications and to capitalize on these insights to discover new therapeutic targets and optimize drug therapy. Such knowledge should make it possible to select drug therapy based on each patient's inherited ability to [respond] to specific medications.
>
> (Evans and Johnson 2001: 11)

Within the realm of the pharmacogenomics endeavour, the genetic variability between individuals confers the ultimate realisation of subject as patient. Through pharmacogenomics, the individual becomes defined in relation to the polymorphisms his or her genetic makeup harbours. The process of subjectivisation is immediately apparent, for, in the molecular attempt to determine interindividual variation, the self becomes the metaphorical equivalent of factors responsible for genetic inheritance, and the subject becomes represented by the charts, figures and graphs that extrapolate on the differences in drug response between individuals. Clinically, pharmacogenomics would ideally eliminate subjects recruited for clinical trials by eliminating those who cannot respond [to drugs] due to inherited differences in drug metabolising enzymes or drug targets (Evans and Johnson 2001: 19).

Pharmacogenomics has undergone a particular evolution with the advent of genomics, and underscores how new technology can directly affect not only the way molecular science is conducted but also the way in which subject formation is intimately related to social organisation through the methods generated by the Human Genome Project. Evans and Johnson highlight the distinction that genomics technology has brought to pharmacogenomics:

The 'pre-genomics' strategy (before 2000) was first to discover an unusual drug response or drug metabolism phenotype, and then to conduct family studies to elucidate inheritance patterns. These steps were followed by cloning of the involved gene and sequencing to identify genotypes that conferred the inherited phenotype. The 'post-genomics' strategy (beginning in 2000) capitalizes on high-throughput sequencing methods and databases generated from the Human Genome Project, to first identify mutations [e.g., single nucleotide polymorphisms (SNPs)], and then search for associations with drug response phenotypes.

(Evans and Johnson 2001: 12)

From the extrapolation from family trees to sequencing the individual genome and searching databases for mutations, the pharmacogenomics strategies transpose the object of study from the social organisation of extended families to the systematic ordering of subjects based on individual genotypes and phenotypes. The variation in drug response is now the product of data mining, rather than deriving from the indirect discovery of genotypes by examining patterns of gene inheritance and through rote cloning.

Ultimately, a secure online database should be developed in which each individual's informative genetic profile will be stored and be available to authorised clinicians (Evans and Johnson 2001: 29). With current technologies, these informative pharmacogenomic phenotypes will likely be determined in panels that are potentially important for their current illness, but with advances in genotyping technology, it should eventually be possible to perform genome-wide detection of hundreds of thousands of informative mutations and to deposit these data well prior to the need to make treatment decisions (Evans and Johnson 2001: 29). The consequent effect on social formations is such that variation in drug response for the explicit aim of optimising medication therapy is a justifiable pretence for classifying individuals according to their genotypes and phenotypes. Individuality now undergirds the teleological imperative for the cataloguing of polymorphisms and their deposition into databases. Subjectivity becomes a construct of genotypic and phenotypic variance.

Interestingly, these examples of technologies emphasise organisation: the organisation of genes in different cell types, the organisation and distribution of chromosomal aberrations, the organisation of gene expression patterns during development and differentiation, and the organisation of genetic polymorphisms into distinct drug response categories. When conceived from a genetic perspective, this emphasis on 'organisation', has enormous implications for subjectivity and social formations, since organisation is an object of both their practices. While organisation seems to be the end result of genomics technology, the individual would be represented according to these norms of organisation. The data from microarray technologies, gene profiling, self-organising maps and the field of pharmacogenomics are organising filters through which the subject could emerge from a potentially fragmented individual to a structured self. As the technology organises data, its results organise society into distinct social formations. In terms of Paul Rabinow's 'biosociality', genomics would produce certain groups organised through treatment plans based on differences in how their neutrophils differentiate, or patients with neurodegenerative diseases forming alliances based on different gene expression waves. The cataloguing of individuals based on their differences in genetic polymorphisms and the elucidation of the polygenetic determinants of drug response and therapy are endeavours in utilising the variation between individuals as a source for organising individuals. Overall, it is the technology of genomics *per se* that is the origin of these instances of biosociality. The organisation of the genome translates into the organisation of the subject and society. Rabinow himself states in the context of biosociality: 'Rather, it is not hard to imagine groups formed around chromosome 17, locus 16,256, site 654,376 allele variant with guanine substitutions. Such groups will have medical specialists, laboratories, narratives, traditions and a heavy panoply of pastoral keepers to help them experience, share and "understand" their fate' (Rabinow 1996). As more complex tests are available, genomics will be used increasingly to classify humans (Hauskeller 2004).

These new data, practices, information and technologies are asking new questions of the ethical subjects of biomedical sciences. These new knowledges have influenced the way that the scientific practices of genomics must now view subjectivity, for it is uniqueness and individuality that is currently at stake. On several levels, the process of subjectivisation is affected. First, individuality becomes tantamount to genetic variance, achieving primacy over other aspects of individual uniqueness. Second, the subject remains uniquely defined by this new notion of the individual. Third, genomics technology and its technical efficiency (aided by databases and computers) ground the subjectivisation process by transforming the individual from subject into patient. This new preconception of the individual as primarily patient is further facilitated by the expected pervasiveness of the HGP technology in all aspects of daily life in the constitution of the subject.

The HGP has revolutionised the way that medicine treats individuality from the perspective of disease and is the progenitor of the conception of the subject as patient. In 'Genetics, biology and disease', Childs and Valle (2000) announce that the HGP promises much in exposing the origins of human individuality: the thousands of genes and their variants that constitute the genetic component of an individuality compounded by experiences of a variable environment through development, maturation and ageing.

We must name and classify diseases, but equally, we should heed the individuality of each patient to whom we give that name. We tend to prefer the name to the individuality, but genetics helps here in revealing the genetic heterogeneity that often explains the diversity and splits off variants, each of which constitutes a new disease with a new name.

(Childs and Valle 2000: 4)

As individual uniqueness is further characterised genetically, the number of diseases will proportionately increase with its commensurate equivalent in new variations of genes. According to the authors, in time the gene products and the homeostatic systems to which they belong will be identified and the participation of their variants in pathogenesis will be characterised (Childs and Valle 2000: 4). In this context, the authors frame the discussion in terms of how differences in allelic combination would lead to variation in the manifestation of diseases:

Further, we shall learn how many of which alleles, derived from how many loci and in how many different combinations, are needed to produce the same disease in different patients, as well as just how the effects of the gene products interact in nonlinear ways to produce variations in clinical expression.

(Childs and Valle 2000: 4)

In the clinical setting this would be equivalent to effecting specific social formations according to the diversity of the clinical expressions of disease:

The HGP will add to the heterogeneity by providing means for further splits and names and there will remain the logistical necessity to group patients for economy of treatment.

(Childs and Valle 2000: 5)

In short, the HGP has revolutionised medical thinking and perspectives on disease itself. In terms of subjectivity, these new notions of disease that the HGP has wrought make explicit the commensuration between individual and patient, mirroring the work of the scientific investigations detailed above.

Yet, questions must be asked of the ethical considerations of the HGP and its technologies and their implications for subjectivity and social formations. Many of our individual features are attributed to the 0.1 per cent (about 3.2 million of the total 3.2 billion) of unshared DNA bases scattered throughout the genome in a location pattern particular to each person. This diversity has been the focus of much research, genetic testing, attempts at commercial exploitation, and concern bordering on fear. Among these implications and issues are the ability to predict future illnesses before any symptoms or medical therapies exist; the privacy and fair use of genetic information with respect to employers, insurers, direct marketers, banks, credit raters, law enforcement agencies, and many others;

the availability of large amounts of genetic information in largely unprotected data banks; and the possible discriminatory misuse of genetic information. One potential (though admittedly extreme) outcome of the HGP is that genome research and the wide use of genetic screening could foster a genetic underclass, leading to a host of new societal conflicts and exacerbating other longstanding divisions (Department of Energy – Ethical, Legal and Social Implications [DOE-ELSI] n.d.).

The ELSI, devoted to understanding and promoting the social implications of the Human Genome Project, deals extensively with these issues. From a social standpoint, the HGP seems to raise a myriad of ethical considerations and caveats to its utilisation and application to society. In terms of purposes of disclosure, the spectre of discrimination in the workplace, and of forensic science, the HGP has raised controversy and the ELSI has documented many studies in promoting education. *However, in the sole instance of exclusively curing disease, genetic information provided by the HGP and its technological corollaries to that objective remains in most cases inviolable.* That is, the uniqueness of the individual remains focused on his or her genetic composition in relation to the diseases that the individual (potentially) harbours. The connection between subjectivity and curing disease should be made explicit. Individuals are no longer human beings foremost; they are patients and may remain subservient to the technological advances of molecular genetics, molecular biology and genomics. The subject becomes subjectivised by these forces of exteriority, and social formations would form in response to the scientific and medical parameters of disease, disorder and illness.

The technologies that I have represented, or the examples of technologies, should not be considered abstractly or placed in a theoretical vault of scientificity. They have discrete effects on organising individuals and effecting social formations, not just in their content but also in their form. They do not obviate the human element in their application. According to Rabinow (1996), we are partially moving from face-to-face surveillance of individuals and groups with the potential to be dangerous or ill toward projecting risk factors that reconstruct the individual or group subject. Monitoring those with genetic predispositions to diabetes, cancer, multiple sclerosis, etc., and discovering them, could be accomplished and involves the likely formation of individual identities arising out of these new truths. Biosociality for Rabinow is, for example, the instance of neurofibromatosis groups whose members meet to share their experiences, lobby for those with disease, educate their children and redo their home environment.

However, what interests me is biosociality in this sense: scientific data is the new progenitor for the human subject, replacing the traditional role ascribed to metaphysics. Rabinow states in a similar fashion that, through the use of computers, individuals sharing certain traits or sets of traits can be grouped together in a way that not only decontextualises them from their social environment but also is nonsubjective in a double sense: it is objectively arrived at, and does not apply to a subject in anything like the older sense of the word (that is, the suffering, meaningfully situated, integrator of social, historical and bodily experiences). Yet this is not exactly the case. The data arising from the HGP technologies *directly apply* to the subject, for they form the practices of exteriority and external forces that integrate the individual, affect his or her suffering, position the subject within a certain framework of social organisation and contextualise the notion of selfhood. While being powered by the efficiency of genomics, the effects of this technology and resulting scientific data on subject formation are all the more magnified. Rabinow asserts that the 'target' of genomics technology (he terms this the 'new genetics') is not a person but a population at risk. However, as diseases become individualised according to particular genotypes and phenotypes, the 'target' of these new scientific constructs is actually the individual. Rabinow's approach simply seems outdated, which may be reflective of the fact that his conception of biosociality predates the genomics era and the advent of the complete sequencing of the human genome.

To understand the implications of this for subjectivity, we must acknowledge that subjectivity has traditionally been considered from a metaphysical standpoint. From Aristotle to St Augustine, to Heidegger and to Foucault, subjectivity has mainly been treated from the perspective of philosophy. Subjectivity is the definitive predicator of an individual's uniqueness. In *Dasein* and *Sein*, subjectivity is inseparable from exteriority. For Descartes, although he never used the word 'subject', we can infer his notion of subjectivity from the thinking and doubting 'I'. However, how much value are we to assign to the notions of subjectivity and the philosophical study of them with the growing predominance of genomics? From a genetic perspective, uniqueness translates as sequence variation and variants and is separable from *Dasein* or *Cogito*. Paradoxically it is an exterior force in the Foucauldian sense, but it reverses the poststructuralist move of the death of the subject. The subject re-emerges from a sea of code; for scientists are not producing data, they are producing subjects.

Our subjective selves may well be dictated by our standards for being a good citizen, a good parent, or a good worker. It may be difficult to admit that individual expression is a manifestation of our template of gene expression. This may indeed be a reduction which is too difficult to accept. It does, however, reinforce the necessity of understanding the Human Genome Project and its associated technologies.

Notes

1 Dr Amanda Orenstein (2004) 'Using microarrays to genotype normal individuals', 1 March, UC Irvine, Irvine, California; personal communication.

References

Barrans, J. D., Ip, J., Lam., C.-W., Hwang, I. L., Dzau, V. J. and Liew, C.-C. (2003) 'Chromosomal distribution of the human cardiovascular transcriptome', *Genomics*, 81: 519–24.

Best, S. (1995) *The Politics of Historical Vision: Marx, Foucault, Habermas*. New York: The Guildford Press Centre for Citizenship, Identity and Governance.

Childs, B. and Valle, D. (2000) 'Genetics, biology and disease', *Annual Review of Genomics and Human Genetics*, 1: 1–19.

Department of Energy-Ethical, Legal and Social Implications (DOE-ELSI) (n.d.) Website: http://www.ornl.gov/sci/techresources/Human_Genome/resource/elsiprog. shtml#intro (accessed 25 July 2006).

Dumur, C. I., Dechsukhum, C., Ware, J. L., Cofield, S. S., Best, A. M., Wilkinson, D. S., Garrett, C. T. and Ferreira-Gonzalez, A. (2003) 'Genome-wide detection in prostate cancer using human SNP microarray technology', *Genomics*, 81: 260–9.

Evans, W. E. and Johnson, J. A. (2001) 'Pharmacogenomics: the inherited basis for interindividual differences in drug response', *Annual Review of Genomics and Human Genetics*, 2: 9–39.

Foucault, M. (1985) *The Use of Pleasure: the history of sexuality*, vol. 2. New York: Random House.

Ge, J., Walhout, A. J. M. and Vidal, M. (2003) 'Integrating "omic" information: A bridge between genomics and systems biology', *Trends in Genetics*, 19: 551–60.

Hauskeller, C. (2004) '*Genes*, genomes and identity: projections on matter', *New Genetics and Society*, 23: 285–99.

Mir, K. U. and Southern, E. M. (2000) 'Sequence variation in genes and genomic DNA: methods for large-scale analysis', *Annual Review of Genomics and Human Genetics*, 1: 329–60.

Rabinow, P. (1996) *Essays on the Anthropology of Reason*. Princeton, NJ: Princeton University Press.

Tamayo, P., Slonim, D., Mesirov, J., Zhu, Q., Kitareewan, S., Dmitrovsky, E., Lander, E. S. and Golub, T. R. (1999) 'Interpreting patterns of gene expression with self-organizing maps: methods and application to hematopoietic differentiation', *Proceedings National Academy of Science USA*, 96: 2907–12.

Vaughan, D. (1996) *To Know Ourselves*. Available online at the ELSI Retrospective Website: http://www.ornl.gov/sci/techresources/HumanGenome/resource/elsiprog. shtml#intro (accessed 25 July 2006).

Wen, X., Fuhrman, S., Michaels, G. S., Carr, D. B., Smith, S., Barker, J. L. and Somogyi, R. (1998) 'Large-scale temporal gene expression mapping of central nervous system development', *Proceedings National Academy of Science USA*, 95: 334–9.

Whitney, A. R., Diehn, M., Popper, S. J., Alizadeh, A. A., Boldrick, J. C., Relman, D. A. and Brown, P. O. (2003): 'Individuality and variation in gene expression patterns in human blood', *Proceedings National Academy of Science USA*, 100: 1896–901.

Index

accountability of patient organisations 31–4
advocacy of patient organisations 39–41, 41–2
Alzheimer's Society 31
ambiguity, genetic knowledge and 141, 142
articulation in public engagement 141

Bauman, Z. 142, 151, 152
behavioural genetics 5, 6
biobanks 21–2
biodiversity, language of 80–81
biogeographical ancestry analysis 78–9, 88, 89–96
biological reductionism 5–7
biomedicine 1, 57, 132, 133; biomedical innovation 1–2, 51; biomedical science 1, 3, 9, 13, 52, 59, 120, 158, 186; post-genomics biomedical research 48; research, potential for 177; technological change and emergence of modern medicine 12
biosocial collectivism 11
biosociality 178, 186, 188–9
biovalue 12, 19–20, 24
blood donors, susceptibility or risk of genetic haemochromatosis in 124–36
Blood of the Vikings (Richards, J.) 7
Butler, Peter 66

Castells, M. 139, 152
categorisation, problem of 144, 178–9
Cavalli-Sforza, Luca 80
CCIG (Centre for Citizenship, Identity and Governance, UK) 179
CESAGen 116, 136
civil society: citizen groups and 149–51
clinical application of genetic testing 47
clinical diagnosis of genetic haemochromatosis 121

computational bioscience 9, 45, 48, 49, 51, 54, 55, 62, 77, 82, 143–4, 186, 188–9
confidentiality: confidential information, disclosure of 167; protection of 21–2
consultation initiatives 147, 152
corporate deployment of science 144
cystic fibrosis, 'geneticisation' of 122

'deep ancestry' 79, 86, 91–2, 96
deliberation, new modes of 30
democracy 35–6
Descartes, René 189
determinism 3–4, 5, 56, 57, 79, 93
diagnostic inference 123
disciplinary boundaries 9, 49, 139, 142
Dutch Parkinsons patients' society (PPV) 32–3, 35, 41
dysmorphology 102–3; absolving parents from blame 107–11; aetiology, explanations of 107–8; clinical management of children 115; ethnographic study of interactional processes 103–16; families and children 111–13; genetic diagnosis, potential of 105; identity work in medical setting 115–16; interpersonal judgements 107; moral and sentimental work 104–7; moral work 113–16; parental surveillance 105–6; personal agency 106–7; reassurance 108–10, 114; research outline 103–4; responsibility 106; sentimental repair work 110–11; stigmatisation 115–16

economies of life 18–20
ELSI (Ethical, Legal and Social Implications) 46, 188
embodiment and 'self' 63–4
embryos, donors of 164–5
entrepreneurial science 142

ESRC (Economic and Social Research Council, UK) 116, 136
ETC group 143, 144, 148
ethics: diversity of ethical views 31; ethical controversy, patient organisations 30–2, 35–6, 38; macroethics 55; of post-genomic science 44–6; subjectivisation and 186–8
eugenics 6
evolutionary psychology 6
experimental organism, perfection in 51–3
expert advice, independence in 142
exteriority and 'society of genomics' 178–9

facial disfigurement 64–7; face transplantation in 65–7
familial risk 3–4
Family Tree DNA 78–9, 88, 89–96, 97–8
fashioning flesh 61–74; aesthetics and economics of fashion 62; elective or essential 63; embodiment and 'self' 63–4; flesh, medicine and fashion 72; genomics and fashion 72–4; latency and 69–70; paradox and conundrum of fashion 67–70; postpartum surgery 65; self-identity and body options 62; technoluxe 62–3; transience of fashion 68–9
Foucault, Michel 1–2, 133, 134, 189; Foucauldian 'techniques of the self' 177–80
Franklin, S. 12, 13, 159, 162

gamete/embryo donors, role of 164–5
gender concerns, reproductive technologies 164–9
gender inequalities 160, 163
gender roles 85–6
gene function 178
GENECLUSTER 182–3
genetic advocacy 8–9; AFM (Association Français contre les Myopathies) 14; biobanks 21–2; biovalue 12, 19–20, 24; bisocial collectivism 11; Coalition of Heritable Disorders of Connective Tissue 18; Genetic Alliance 18; genetic diseases, hope, identity and governance of 15–18; genetic support groups 18–19; groups 11–24; hope, capitalisation, relational qualities of 13; hope, vision and 16–17, 23–4; Human Genome Project (HGP) 11; IVF (*in vitro* fertilisation) 13; markets, morals and values 21–2; National Institutes of Health (US) 18; participatory role of 14, 16, 17, 20, 22; patent licensing 20;

Patient Advocates for Skin Disease Research 18; patients groups, growth of 13–14; political advocacy 18, 22–3; political economies of hope 11, 12–15; PXE International 12, 14, 15–18, 21, 22; Blood and Tissue Bank 19–20; scientific knowledge, production of 14, 16, 17, 20; wealth creation 20
Genetic Alliance 18
genetic ancestry tracing 86–8
genetic body 46–8
genetic choices, prioritisation of 147–8
genetic diagnostics 147–8
genetic difference, gradients of 83
genetic diseases, hope, identity and governance of 15–18
genetic distinctions, advances in determination of 178–9
genetic genealogy 88–96
genetic haemochromatosis 120–36; clinical diagnosis of 121; cystic fibrosis, 'geneticisation' of 122; diagnostic inference 123; experiences of 121–2, 123–4, 126–32, 132–3; geneticisation of contemporary medicine 122–3; HFE gene, discovery of 120–21; identification of susceptibility or risk in blood-donors study 124–36; ambiguity in clinical encounters 130–32; classification and experience 132–4; diagnosis, difficulties with 128–9, 132; disease features 126; fieldwork 125; interviews with patients 125–6; non-specific symptoms 128–30; nosography of haemochromatosis 126–32, 133–4; research outline 124–6; subjects 125–6; symptoms, divergent nature of 126–7, 128–9; uncertainty in clinical encounters 130–32; lay phenomenology of 122; prediction of 121; susceptibility to 121, 122
genetic ignorance of geographical origins 79
genetic life chances 147–8
genetic lineage, passages of 83
genetic polymorphisms 183–4, 186
genetic reductionism 5–6
genetic risk 3–4
genetic screening 47, 147–8
genetic support groups 18–19
genetic syndromes *see* dysmorphology
genetic therapies, fashion and 68–9, 72–4
genetic uniqueness, methodological organisation of 184–5
geneticisation 4–5; of contemporary medicine 122–3
genetics 1, 4, 7; behavioural genetics 5, 6; contemporary genetics 6, 11–23;

ethical and social issues in 9; gender and reproductive technologies in Latin America 157–71; new genetics 11–23; reproductive technologies and 9, 157–73; *see also* genetic advocacy, groups; genetic haemochromatosis; genetic syndromes; genomics; mapping origins; patient organisations; post-genomics; public engagement
'Genetics, Biology and Disease' 186–7
Genewatch 147
Genographic Project, The 8, 77–9, 80–88, 96–8
genomics 1; biosociality 178, 186, 188–9; bodily transformations, 'fashioning flesh' 61–74; ELSI (Ethical, Legal and Social Implications) 189; ethics and subjectivisation 186–8; exteriority and 'society of genomics' 178–9; fashion and 61, 72–4; fluidity of genomic science 143–4; Foucauldian 'techniques of the self' 177–8, 179–80; gene function 178; GENECLUSTER 182–3; genes 178; genetic distinctions, advances in determination of 178–9; genetic polymorphisms 183–4, 186; genetic uniqueness; genomic innovations 143–4, 148; GM initiatives and 149; green genomics 147; heterozygosity, loss of (LOH) 180–1, 182; Human Genome Project (HGP) 177, 178, 183–9; identities, concept of 179; identities, government and 148–9; identities, poststructuralist approaches to 179; identities, subjectivity and 178; individuality, genetic variance and 186–7; interindividual variation in peripheral blood cells 180; microarrays 183; pharmacogenomics 183–5; philosophy, molecular science and 177; potential for biomedical research 177; proteins 178; red genomics 147; self-organising maps 182–3; social formations and disease expressions 187–8; social organisation, impacts on 182–3; societal implications, far reaching 177; subjectivity 177–8, 182–3, 188–9; genomics technologies and 179; teleology of 177; temporal gene expression in the CNS 181–2
GM Nation? 150
groups, genetic advocacy of 11–24

Habermas, Jürgen 140–41, 143, 147, 149–50, 153–4
Haraway, D. J. 45, 77, 80, 88, 122, 134

healthcare system, major players 28
heterozygosity, loss of (LOH) 180–1, 182
HFE gene, discovery of 120–21
hope: capitalisation through biomedics 13; political economies of 11, 12–15; relational qualities of 13; vision and 16–17, 23–4
Horizon 149
human diversity, maps of 84–5
Human Genome Diversity Project (HGDP) 80–88
Human Genome Project (HGP) 3; genetic advocacy 11; genomics, social formations and the 177, 178, 183–9
human organism, molecular biology of 44–58; clinical application of genetic testing 47; complexity, predictability and 56; ELSI (Ethical, Legal and Social Implications) 46, 188; ethics of post-genomic science 44–6; experimental organism, perfection in 51–3; genetic body 46–8; genetic screening 47; Human Genome Project (HGP) 46–7; macroethics 55; molecular descriptions of biological processes 44, 45; molecular intervention 48; National Human Genome Institute (NHGRI, US) 45, 46, 50; Physiome Project 54–5; post-genomic bioethics 48–9; post-genomic biomedical research 48; post-genomic bodies, construction of 45–6; post-genomic body 48–51; post-genomic knowledge production 49; post-genomic technologies 49; post-genomic visions 51–6; predictability, promise of 50, 56; research relationships 45; social consequences of genetic information 47–8, 53; social relations, technoscience and 44–5; stabilisation 50–51; systems and risk 54–5; Systems Biology 50–51; systems innovation 45; systems-level science, convergence towards 49–50; systems nature of post-genomic science 49–51, 53–6, 57; virtual predictive organism 53–6

identities: 'Black Jews' 7; collective identity 7, 8; concept of 179; gender identity 179; gendered identity 146; national and biological, intersection of 7–8; post-structuralist approaches to 179; social identities 142; subjectivity and 178
independent expert advice 142

individuality, genetic variance and 186–7
informed consent 165–6
inheritance 3–4
innovation 1, 57, 72, 159, 178;
    biomedical innovation 1–2, 51;
    genomic innovations 143–4, 148;
    innovation policy 29; innovation
    processes 44–5, 142; markets
    innovation 169; in plastic surgery 66;
    relevance for self-identity 1–2; social
    innovation 152; systems innovation
    45; technological innovation 45, 48–9,
    56, 151, 153, 181
Institute for Stem Cell Research 39–40
institutions, interdisciplinarity and
    143–5
interactional processes in dysmorphology
    clinic 103–16; absolving parents from
    blame 107–10; clinical management of
    children 115; confessional space 104;
    families and children 111–13; genetic
    diagnosis 105; identity work in
    medical setting 115–16; interpersonal
    judgements 107; moral and sentimental
    work 104–7; moral attributions 106;
    moral work 113–16; parental
    surveillance 105–6; personal agency
    106–7; reassurance 108–10, 114;
    research outline 103–4; responsibility
    106; sentimental repair work 110–11;
    stigmatisation 115–16
interdisciplinarity 9–10, 46, 49, 54, 142
interindividual variation in peripheral
    blood cells 181
international studies, reproductive
    technologies 158–60
IVF (*in vitro* fertilisation): genetic
    advocacy 13; patient organisations 30

Kant, Immanuel 67, 68
knowledge: genetic knowledge and
    ambiguity 141, 142; history of
    biomedical knowledge 6; open-source
    knowledge 144; post-genomic
    knowledge production 49; production
    of scientific knowledge 14, 16, 17, 20;
    social robustness of scientific
    knowledge 30

Latin American Network on Assisted
    Reproduction (LARA) 63, 163, 167
Latour, Bruno 48
legitimacy for patient organisations 29–30,
    31–2, 35–6
life sciences 19, 20, 45, 50, 56, 171
linking with patients 37–8, 41–2

macroethics 55
Manifesto of the Cyborg 134
mapping origins 77–98; biogeographical
    ancestry analysis 78–9, 88, 89–96; 'deep
    ancestry' 79, 86, 91–2, 96; Family Tree
    DNA 78–9, 88, 89–96, 97–8; genetic
    ancestry tracing 86–8; genetic difference,
    gradients of 83; genetic genealogy
    88–96; genetic ignorance of geographical
    origins 79; Genographic Project 77–9,
    80–8, 96–8; human diversity, maps of
    84–5; Human Genome Diversity Project
    (HGDP) 80–8; migration and genetic
    interconnection 81; mitochondrial
    DNA 83, 89–90, 92, 93, 95, 96;
    National Geographic Society 77;
    Oxford Ancestors 95; passages of
    genetic lineage 83; political
    considerations 86; population genetics
    80–88; 'populations' and 'groups' 83–4;
    preservation of human diversity 80–1;
    Relative Genetics 88–9; similarity,
    language of 82; Waitt Family
    Foundation 77, 82–3; Wells' 'Journey
    of Man' 81–2, 86; Y-DNA 83, 87, 89,
    90, 92, 93, 94, 96
markets: drug markets 50; genealogical
    market 78; health services in Europe
    163; market forces 141, 154; market
    relations 21; market values 144;
    marketing genetic tests 89, 92, 94, 95,
    97; markets innovation 169; morals
    and values 21–2; neo-liberal market
    logic 148
Melucci, A. 139, 147, 151
microarrays 182–4
migration and genetic interconnection 81
mitochondrial DNA 83, 89–90, 92, 93,
    95, 96
molecular descriptions of biological
    processes 44, 45
molecular intervention 48
morality and genomic techniques 141
motherhood, changes in notions of 168–70
multidisciplinary collaboration 104, 124–5

National Geographic Society 77
National Human Genome Institute
    (NHGRI, US) 45, 46, 50
National Institutes of Health (US) 18
networked social milieu 139, 147
Nielsen, Linda 145

open-source knowledge 144
organisation, emphasis on 185–6
Oxford Ancestors 95

Parkinson Disease Society (PDS) 31–2, 33, 35, 41
participatory role in genetic advocacy 14, 16, 17, 20, 22
Patenting Human Genes and Stem Cells (Danish Council of Ethics) 145
patents: patent licensing 20; patenting medical genetics 145–6
Patient Advocates for Skin Disease Research 18
patient organisations 8–9, 28–42; accountability 31–4; advocacy of 39–41, 41–2; Alzheimer's Society 31; deliberation, new modes of 30; democracy 35–6; Diabetes UK 31; diversity of ethical views 31; Dutch Parkinsons patients' society (PPV) 32–3, 35, 41; establishment of 28; ethical controversy 30–32, 35–6, 38; Institute for Stem Cell Research 39–40; legitimacy 29–30, 31–2, 35–6; linking with patients 37–8, 41–2; major players in healthcare system 28; Parkinson Disease Society (PDS) 31–2, 33, 35, 41; patients' groups, growth of 13–14; political role 28–9; presentation of proof 38–41; 'public' and 'community' 36–8; public disputes, role in 29; 'public good' 35; representation in politics 33–6; representation of patients 36–8, 41–2; scientific knowledge, social robustness of 30; self-assuredness of 33; stem cell research 30–31, 33; therapeutic cloning 30–31
PDS (Parkinson's Disease Society) 31–2, 35, 38–9, 41
peripheral blood cells, interindividual variation in 180
pharmacogenomics 183–5
philosophy 69, 73, 124, 141, 189; molecular science and 177; moral philosophy 170; political philosophy 36
policy recommendations, reproductive technologies in Latin America 170–1
political advocacy 18, 22–3
political considerations in mapping origins 86
political economies of hope 11, 12–15
political representation of patient organisations 33–6
political role of patient organisations 28–9
population genetics 80–88
'populations' and 'groups', mapping origins 83–4
post-genomics: bioethics of 48–9; biomedical research 48; body and

being of 48–51; knowledge production 49; organisations, construction of 45–6; science 6, 9; systems nature of 49–51, 53–6, 57; technologies 49; visions 51–6
postpartum surgery 65
PPV (Dutch Parkinsons Patients Society) 32–3, 35, 41
predictability: prediction of genetic haemochromatosis 121; promise of 50, 56
pregnancy, changes in notions of 167–69
presentation of proof by patient organisations 38–41
preservation of human diversity 80–81
proteins 178
proto-politics, emergence of 140–41
public acceptability of scientific developments 140
'public' and 'community' organisations 36–8
public awareness of reproductive technologies 167–8
public disputes, patient organisations' role in 29
public engagement 9, 139–54; ambiguity, genetic knowledge and 141, 142; articulation of 141; categorisation, problem of 144; civil society, citizen groups and 149–51; civil society, social movements and 147–8; collective stakes 147; computational bioscience 143; consultation initiatives, difficulty of finding respondents 147; copyright licensing 146; corporate deployment of science 144; disciplinary boundaries 139; disciplinary identities 142; entrepreneurial science 142; fluidity of genomic science 143–4; genetic choices, prioritisation of 147–8; genetic diagnostics 147–8; genetic life chances 147–8; Genewatch 147; genomics, GM initiatives and 149; genomics, identity and government 148–9; green genomics 147; Greenpeace 147; independent expert advice 142; institutions, interdisciplinarity and 143–5; morality and genomic techniques 141; networked social milieu 139, 147; open-source knowledge 144; patenting 145–6; proto-politics, emergence of 140–41; proto-politics of genomics 140; public acceptability of scientific developments 140; red genomics 147; seeds of 139; self-identity of scientists 142; social actors and institutions 139–40; social anatomy

142; social and moral risk 140; social
identities 142
'public good' 34–5
PXE International 12, 14, 15–18, 21, 22;
Blood and Tissue Bank 19–20

Rabinow, Paul 7, 14, 15, 23, 24, 47, 178,
186, 188–9
regional studies, reproductive
technologies in Latin America 158–60
Relative Genetics 88–9
reproductive technologies in Latin
America: confidential information,
disclosure of 167; discourse and
practices 160–2; embryos, use of 164–5;
ethical concerns 164–8; follow-up
procedures 167; gamete/embrio donors,
role of 164–5; gender concerns 164–8;
informed consent 165–6; international
studies 158–60; motherhood, changes
in notions of 168–70; policy
recommendations 170–1; pregnancy,
changes in notions of 168–70; public
awareness 167–8; record-keeping 167;
regional studies 158–60; social concerns
164–8; trends in NRTs 162–4
risk 5, 11, 14, 17, 41, 45, 47, 51, 184,
188–9; of congenital malformation
166; familial risk 3–4; genetic risk 3–4,
47, 53, 120, 135; predictive risk 53; in
reproductive technologies 160, 162,
164, 166, 170; risk assessment 2;
scientific and professional
identification of 2–3; social and moral
risk 140; systems and risk 54–5

Sanger Institute 143, 144
science: biomedical science 1, 3, 9, 13,
52, 59, 120, 158, 186; life sciences 19,
20, 45, 50, 56, 171; popular science
6–7; production of scientific
knowledge 14, 16, 17, 20; social
robustness of scientific knowledge 30;
and technology 29, 140, 169
Science and Technology, House of Lords
Select Committee on 30
self: embodiment and 'self' 63–4;
self-assuredness of patient organisations
33; self-identity and body options 62;
self-identity of scientists 142
self-organising maps 182–3
Seven Daughters of Eve, The 7, 92, 95
Shriver, M. and Kittles, R. 78, 92, 93
social actors and institutions 139–40
social anatomy 142
social and moral risk 140

social concerns, reproductive
technologies 164–8
social consequences of genetic
information 47–8, 53
social formations 1; and disease
expressions 187–8
social identities 1, 142; biological
expression of 6
social implications of genomics 177
social innovation 151
social milieu 139, 147
social organisation, genomics impact on
182–3
social relations, technoscience and 44–5
social sciences 5, 6, 24, 150, 159, 171
Staal, J. 33
stabilisation in molecular biology 50–1
stem cell research 30–1, 33
stem cell technologies 5
stigmatisation 4, 8, 18, 102, 110,
115–16, 158, 167
subjectivity 177–8, 182–3, 188–9;
genomics technologies and 179
systems and risk 54–5
Systems Biology 50–51
systems innovation 45
systems-level science, convergence
towards 49–50
systems nature of post-genomic science
49–51, 53–6, 57

technological innovation 45, 48–9, 56,
151, 153, 181
technoluxe 62–3
teleology of genomics 177
temporal gene expression in the CNS
181–2
theodicy of suffering 3–4
therapeutic cloning 30–31
tissue engineering 6

UNESCO 157
US National Human Genome Institute
(NHGRI) 45, 50
virtual predictive organism 53–6
VSOP, Netherlands 29

Waitt Family Foundation 77, 82–3
Waldby, Catherine 2, 12, 19, 122
wealth creation 20
Wells, Spencer 77, 81–2, 86; 'Journey of
Man' 81–2, 86
Wynne, B. 49, 140, 146

Y-DNA (Y-chromosome) 83, 87, 89, 90,
92, 93, 94, 96

For Product Safety Concerns and Information please contact our EU
representative GPSR@taylorandfrancis.com
Taylor & Francis Verlag GmbH, Kaufingerstraße 24, 80331 München, Germany

www.ingramcontent.com/pod-product-compliance
Ingram Content Group UK Ltd.
Pitfield, Milton Keynes, MK11 3LW, UK
UKHW021121180425
457613UK00005B/173